WEIGHT LOSS DIET COOKBOOK FOR SENIOR CITIZENS

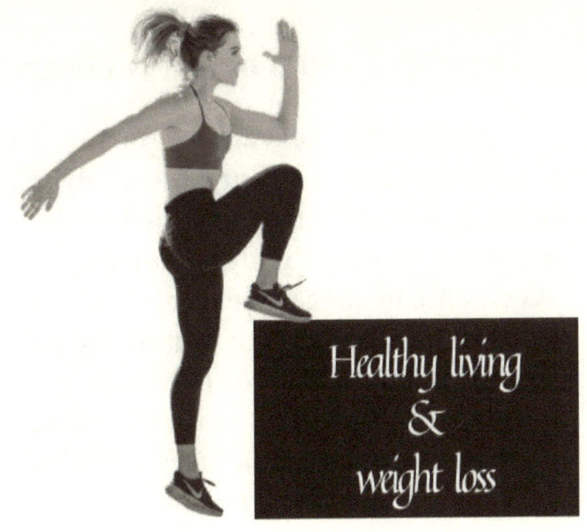

Nourishing Your Wellness Journey, Savor the Flavors of Health and Longevity

Lucas Livingston

Table of Contents

- **Main Course Meals**
- **Snacks and Treats**
- **Desserts for a Sweet Treat**

Managing Diabetes and Blood Sugar

- **Heart Health and Hypertension**
- **Weight Management for Seniors**
- **Joint and Bone Health**
- **Promoting Mental Well-being**

The Importance of Senior Fitness

- **Low-Impact Exercises for Seniors**
- **Yoga and Stretching for Flexibility**
- **Incorporating Physical Activity into Daily Life**

Stress Reduction and Relaxation Techniques

INTRODUCTION

Welcome to the Weight Loss Diet for Seniors

In the golden years of life, the pursuit of health takes center stage. For those who have graced their 60th year and beyond, the importance of a vibrant, fulfilling existence cannot be overstated. It is a chapter of life where we seek not only longevity but also the ability to savor each moment to its fullest.

Enter the Weight Loss Diet—a transformative approach to nutrition and well-being that is tailored to the unique needs of seniors. In the following pages, we embark on a journey that transcends the ordinary boundaries of dieting; we embark on a path toward prolonged vitality and enriched living.

As we age, our bodies undergo remarkable changes. Metabolism slows, energy levels can wane, and health concerns may arise. Yet, within these changes lies an opportunity—an opportunity to reclaim our health, to bolster our resilience, and to embrace each day with renewed vigor.

The Weight Loss Diet for Seniors is not just a diet; it's a philosophy—a philosophy rooted in the belief that age should never be a barrier to experiencing the full spectrum of life's joys. It is a celebration of wholesome, nourishing foods that provide the fuel for vibrant living. It is a tribute to the body's astounding capacity for rejuvenation and self-healing.

In the chapters that follow, we will delve into the core principles of the Weight Loss Diet, explore the art of mindful eating, and discover how the foods we choose can empower us to lead our best lives as seniors. We'll provide you with practical guidance on meal planning, delicious recipes tailored to your needs, and insights into managing specific health concerns that may accompany aging.

But this journey is not limited to the kitchen. We will also explore the significance of staying active, nurturing mental well-being, and fostering a sense of belonging and purpose. It's a holistic approach to aging—one that recognizes that a healthy life is a multi-faceted tapestry, woven with nutrition, exercise, social connection, and the pursuit of passions.

The pages that follow are your guide to unlocking the potential for vibrant health and longevity that resides within you. Together, we'll embark on a transformative journey—one that honors the wisdom of age and harnesses the power of nutrition and lifestyle to ensure that your senior years are not merely endured but celebrated. Welcome to the Weight Loss Diet for Seniors—a path to wellness, vitality, and a life well-lived.

Understanding the Weight Loss Diet Philosophy

Welcome to the transformative journey of understanding the Weight Loss Diet

Philosophy, a path towards holistic well-being and enduring vitality. In a world brimming with fad diets and fleeting health trends, the Weight Loss Diet stands as a beacon of enduring wisdom, designed not merely to help you shed pounds but to rewrite the story of your life beyond 60.

Imagine a lifestyle that celebrates the wisdom of your years, acknowledging the unique nutritional needs and health aspirations that come with age. The Weight Loss Diet is not just another diet plan; it's a profound shift in perspective, a philosophy rooted in the belief that you deserve to enjoy every chapter of your life to the fullest.

As seniors, you've gathered a lifetime of experiences, and now it's time to craft a legacy of health and vitality. The Weight Loss Diet Philosophy centers on simplicity, balance, and nourishing your body, ensuring that each meal is a symphony of taste and nutrition. It's about embracing real, wholesome foods that become your allies in the pursuit of a longer, healthier life.

But this journey is not solely about what you put on your plate. It's a holistic approach that recognizes the interplay between nutrition, physical activity, mental well-being, and the beautiful tapestry of your life experiences. It's about savoring every bite, nurturing your body with love, and reclaiming the vibrancy that's rightfully yours.

In the pages that follow, you'll discover the core principles of the Weight Loss Diet Philosophy, which will empower you to take charge of your health and redefine aging. It's about living a life that's not just longer, but one that's filled with energy, joy, and the freedom to embrace all that life offers. The journey begins here, where your story continues, and where the Weight Loss Diet Philosophy becomes your compass on the path to a healthier, happier you.

Benefits of the Weight Loss Diet for Senior Health

In the graceful tapestry of life, the golden years should be a time of wisdom, serenity, and cherished moments. Yet, for many seniors, health challenges can cast shadows on this beautiful phase. Enter the Weight Loss Diet, a beacon of hope, a guide to longevity, and a recipe for vibrant senior living.

1. Blood Sugar Mastery:

Seniors often grapple with fluctuating blood sugar levels, a concern that can undermine vitality. The Weight Loss Diet, with its balanced approach to carbohydrates, reignites control over blood sugar. It offers a lifeline, reducing the risk of diabetes complications and providing newfound energy for cherished pursuits.

2. Weight Wellness:

Weight management becomes pivotal as the years roll by, and the Weight Loss Diet understands this intimately. Tailored for seniors, it encourages gradual, sustainable weight loss through wholesome nutrition.

Shedding excess pounds becomes a gentle journey, alleviating strain on aging joints and nurturing heart health.

3. Heartfelt Protection:

The beat of life resonates within our hearts, and the Weight Loss Diet safeguards this precious organ. With its emphasis on heart-healthy choices, such as lean proteins, fiber-rich foods, and antioxidants, it fortifies the cardiovascular system, ushering seniors toward the promise of more heartbeats, more laughter, and more cherished moments.

4. Nutrient Abundance:

Nutrition often takes center stage in senior health, and the Weight Loss Diet offers a feast of essential nutrients. It celebrates fresh fruits, vibrant vegetables, and whole grains, fortifying the body with vitamins, minerals, and antioxidants. Seniors thrive on this nutritional bounty, their bodies celebrating every delicious bite.

5. Digestive Ease:

The Weight Loss Diet understands that aging can bring digestive challenges. It eases this journey with its fiber-rich approach, promoting regularity and digestive comfort. Seniors find solace in meals that nourish not just the body but the intricate workings of the digestive system.

6. Mental Clarity:

The mind is a treasure trove of memories and wisdom, and the Weight Loss Diet is a guardian of mental clarity. Through the power of balanced nutrition, it nurtures brain health, enhancing cognitive function. Seniors revel in the joy of sharp thinking and remain active participants in life's adventures.

7. Active Living:

The Weight Loss Diet is a key that unlocks the door to active living. With balanced meals that fuel the body, seniors rediscover the joys of movement. Whether it's gentle yoga, a leisurely stroll, or a dance in the living room, the Weight Loss Diet breathes life into every step and gesture.

In the journey of life, age is but a number, and the Weight Loss Diet is a timeless companion. It empowers seniors to savor each moment, cherish their health, and embrace the beauty of longevity. With blood sugar tamed, hearts fortified, and minds sharpened, seniors become the authors of their own vibrant stories, living life to the fullest. Welcome to the Weight Loss Diet - where health and vitality know no bounds, and the golden years truly shine.

Eternal Vitality: Nina's Journey to 120 Years of Health and Happiness with the Weight loss Diet.

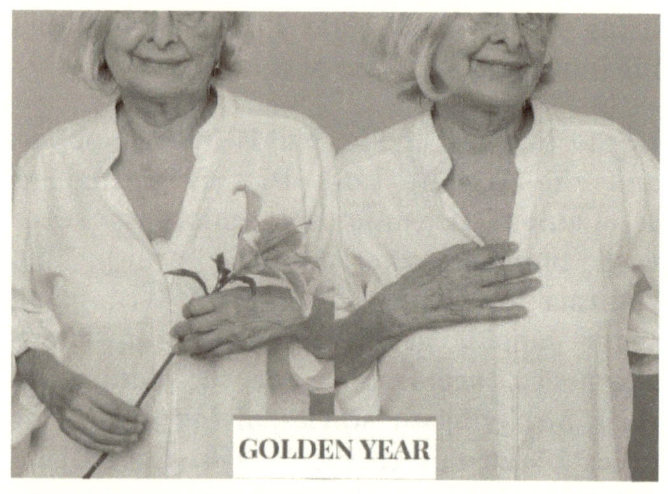

Nina had always been a woman of great determination and a zest for life. As she approached her 60th birthday, she couldn't help but reflect on the passing years and her health. Despite her active lifestyle and relatively healthy eating habits, the specter of aging loomed large in her mind. She had seen friends and family members struggle with various health issues, and she was determined to find a way to ensure her own longevity.

One sunny morning, while sipping her tea and scrolling through the latest health news online, Nina stumbled upon an article that caught her eye - "Nourishing Your Wellness Journey,Savor the Flavors of Health and Longevity" by Lucas Livingston. Intrigued by the promise of a longer, healthier life, she dove headfirst into researching the Weight Loss Diet.

The Weight Loss Diet, she discovered, was not just another fad. It was a comprehensive and sustainable approach to weight management and overall health. Unlike other diets,it focused on balancing insulin levels to optimize metabolism, control blood sugar, and promote fat loss. It emphasized whole foods, portion control, and regular exercise as part of a holistic lifestyle change.

Nina decided to give it a try. She started by cleaning out her pantry, replacing processed foods with whole grains, lean proteins, and an abundance of colorful fruits and vegetables. She also began practicing mindful eating, savoring every bite and appreciating the nourishment her body received.

As the weeks turned into months, Nina experienced remarkable changes. Her energy levels soared, and her cravings for sugary snacks disappeared. She started shedding excess weight effortlessly, and her blood sugar levels stabilized. Nina was astounded by how good she felt, both physically and mentally.

With her newfound vitality, Nina embraced a more active lifestyle. She took up yoga and began walking daily, relishing the simple joy of being outdoors. She also made it a point to prioritize rest and relaxation, practicing meditation to reduce stress and boost her overall well-being.

Years passed, and Nina celebrated her 80th birthday with a vitality that defied her age. Her friends and family marveled at her youthful spirit and radiant health. She continued to follow the Weight Loss Diet principles faithfully, and her annual check-ups with her doctor consistently yielded stellar results. Her doctor often joked that

Nina was a living testament to the benefits of a balanced and mindful approach to eating.

Nina's 100th birthday was a grand affair, attended by friends and family from all over the world. She stood before them, still spry and full of life, and credited her long and healthy life to the Weight Loss Diet. Her story had inspired many to adopt healthier lifestyles, and she had become a local legend.

As the years rolled on, Nina's health remained robust. She danced at her great-grandchildren's weddings, hiked in the mountains, and even took up painting as a new hobby. At 120 years old, she was a living testament to the power of the Weight Loss Diet and the determination to live life to its fullest.

Nina's story spread far and wide, becoming a symbol of hope and inspiration for generations to come. She proved that with the right mindset and a commitment to a balanced, healthy lifestyle, age could be just a number, and life could be lived to its fullest potential.

Getting Started: Tips for Success

As we age, our bodies undergo incredible transformations, and maintaining optimal health becomes a precious pursuit. Enter the Weight Loss Diet, a powerful and proven approach designed specifically for seniors above 60. It's not just a diet; it's a lifestyle that empowers you to take control of your health and savor the joys of aging gracefully. Here are some invaluable tips to kickstart your journey towards a healthier, happier you:

1. Embrace the Weight Loss Diet Philosophy: Understand that the Weight Loss Diet isn't just about shedding pounds; it's about nourishing your body, stabilizing blood sugar, and enhancing your overall well-being. Embrace this holistic approach to senior health.

2.Try to Set Realistic Goals: Define what success really means to you. Whether it's more energy, better blood sugar control, or a slimmer waistline, setting achievable goals will keep you motivated on this path.

3. Educate Yourself: Knowledge is your ally. Take the time to learn about the Weight Loss Diet principles, the foods that support your health, and the ones to avoid. Arm yourself with information to make informed choices.

4. Plan Your Meals: Create a weekly meal plan that's not only delicious but also nutritious. Ensure it includes a variety of fruits, vegetables, lean proteins, and whole grains. Consult Weight Loss Diet recipes for inspiration.

5. Portion Control: As a senior, your portion sizes matter. Be mindful of how much you eat and avoid overindulging. Smaller, balanced portions can work wonders for your health.

6. Stay Hydrated: Dehydration can exacerbate health issues. Make it a habit to

drink plenty of water throughout the day. Hydration is key to feeling your best.

7. Be Patient and Persistent: Rome wasn't built in a day, and neither is vibrant senior health. Understand that results may take time, and setbacks may happen. Stay committed, and don't let momentary lapses derail your journey.

8. Lean on Support: Enlist the support of loved ones or join a Weight Loss Diet community.The sharing of your goals and progress with others can provide motivation and accountability.

9. Prioritize Physical Activity: Even gentle exercises like walking, yoga, or swimming can make a significant difference in your well-being. Aim for regular, low-impact physical activity to keep your body agile.

10. Celebrate Small Wins: Acknowledge and celebrate every achievement, no matter how minor it may seem. Every step forward is a step towards a healthier, happier you.

The Weight Loss Diet is your key to unlocking the door to prolonged health, vitality, and joy in your senior years. Remember, this is not just about the destination; it's about the journey. With dedication, knowledge, and a positive attitude, you have the power to make your golden years truly golden. Your path to vibrant health starts today, and we're here to support you every step of the way. Welcome to a healthier, happier you with the Weight Loss Diet for seniors.

Chapter 1: Senior Nutrition Essentials

Nutrient Needs for Seniors

•Portion Control and Balanced Meals

In today's fast-paced world, maintaining a healthy diet can often feel like a Herculean task. With tempting fast food options on every corner and portion sizes that seem to grow with each passing year, it's no wonder that many of us struggle with weight management and overall health. However, the solution to these modern-day dietary

challenges lies in a simple yet powerful concept: portion control and balanced meals.

Portion control is the art of moderating the amount of food we eat during a single meal or snack. It's not about depriving ourselves, but rather about understanding the right quantity to nourish our bodies without overindulging. When we master portion control, we empower ourselves to make healthier choices and maintain a harmonious relationship with food.

But portion control alone is not enough. Equally important is the composition of our meals. A balanced meal is one that provides us with a diverse range of nutrients to fuel our bodies effectively. It combines essential components, such as carbohydrates, proteins, healthy fats, vitamins, and minerals, in the right proportions. This holistic approach to eating ensures that we meet our nutritional needs while keeping calorie intake in check.

MEAL MAXIMIZATION FOR SENIORS

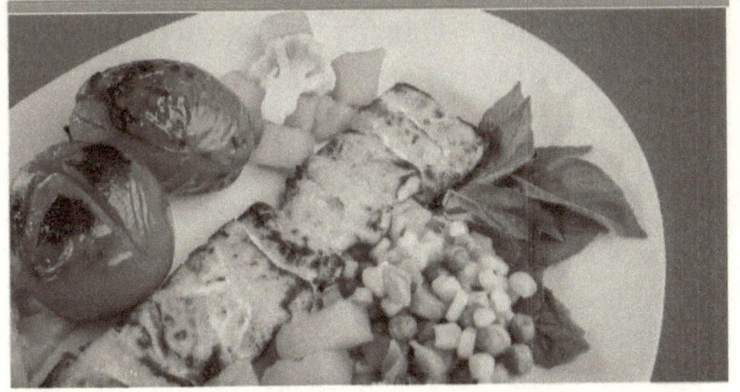

Here's why portion control and balanced meals are so powerful:

- **Weight Management: Portion control helps us avoid excessive calorie consumption, making it an effective tool for weight management. When we eat mindfully and in appropriate amounts, we're more likely to achieve and maintain a healthy weight.**
- **Blood Sugar Control: Balanced meals, with the right mix of carbohydrates, proteins, and fats, help regulate blood**

sugar levels. This is crucial for individuals with diabetes and beneficial for everyone in preventing energy crashes and mood swings.

- Nutrient Density: Balanced meals provide a wealth of essential nutrients, which support overall health. From calcium for strong bones to antioxidants for cellular protection, a variety of nutrients are required for our bodies to function optimally.
- Sustained Energy: Proper portion control and balanced meals provide sustained energy throughout the day. This reduces the temptation to snack on unhealthy options and helps us stay productive and alert.
- Digestive Health: Smaller, well-proportioned meals are easier for the digestive system to handle. Such can alleviate issues like bloating and indigestion.
- Long-Term Wellness: Adopting portion control and balanced eating as a lifestyle choice promotes long-term wellness. It's not a restrictive diet but

a sustainable way to nourish our bodies and enjoy a wide variety of foods.

So, how can we incorporate portion control and balanced meals into our lives?

Start by listening to your body's hunger cues. Eat when you're hungry and stop when you're satisfied, not overly full. Utilize smaller plates to help control portion sizes visually. Aim at filling half your plate with colorful fruits and vegetables, a quarter with lean proteins, and the remaining quarter with whole grains or other complex carbohydrates. Incorporate healthy fats like avocados, nuts, and olive oil into your meals.

Remember that the journey to better health through portion control and balanced meals is a gradual one. This is about making small, sustainable changes to your eating habits. Seek support from a registered dietitian or nutritionist if needed, and embrace the power of mindfulness when it comes to what, when, and how much you eat.

Portion control and balanced meals are not just about the food on your plate; they are about taking control of your health and well-being. By adopting these principles, you can achieve a healthier, happier, and more vibrant life—one balanced bite at a time.

Hydration for Optimal Health

Water, the elixir of life, is often underestimated in its significance. Yet, proper hydration is the cornerstone of optimal health, a silent hero that supports every facet of our well-being. In this comprehensive exploration, we delve into the profound importance of hydration, unveiling its transformative effects on our bodies and minds.

The Body's Vital Fluid:

At its core, our body is a complex network of cells, tissues, and organs, all intricately interconnected. Water plays an irreplaceable role in maintaining this balance. It serves as a transport medium for nutrients, aids in digestion, regulates body temperature, and enables waste elimination. Hi, it is our body's lifeline.

The Daily Requirement:

The recommended daily intake of water varies depending on factors such as age, sex, activity level, and climate. A general guideline is to consume at least eight 8-ounce glasses of water a day, known as the "8x8" rule. However, individual needs may differ, and it's crucial to listen to your body.

Hydration and Physical Health:

Hydration is essential for optimal physical performance. Dehydration, even at mild levels, can lead to fatigue, muscle cramps, and decreased endurance. It hinders the body's ability to cool itself, potentially resulting in heat-related illnesses. Adequate water intake is also crucial for maintaining healthy skin, joints, and organs.

Cognitive Clarity:

Our brain, which comprises about 75% water, depends on proper hydration to function optimally. Dehydration can lead to impaired concentration, memory problems, and mood swings. Staying well-hydrated enhances mental clarity, alertness, and cognitive performance.

Weight Management:

Hydration plays an underestimated role in weight management. Often, our bodies tend to confuse thirst with hunger, leading to unnecessary calorie consumption. By staying hydrated, we can better differentiate between these sensations and reduce overeating.

Detoxification and Immune Support:

Water is instrumental in flushing out toxins and waste products from the body. Adequate hydration supports the kidneys and liver in their detoxification processes. Additionally, it helps bolster the immune system, as it aids in the circulation of white blood cells and antibodies throughout the body.

Aging Gracefully:

Proper hydration can promote healthier aging. It aids in maintaining joint flexibility, reducing the risk of kidney stones, and preventing urinary tract infections – common concerns as we grow older.

Practical Tips for Hydration:

- Carry a reusable water bottle to make it convenient to sip throughout the day.
- Monitor your urine color – pale yellow is a good indicator of adequate hydration.
- The incorporate hydrating foods like fruits and vegetables into your diet.
- Adjust the intake of water based on activity level and climate.

- Be very mindful of caffeine and alcohol intake, as they can contribute to dehydration.

Special Considerations for Aging Digestive Systems

As the years advance, our bodies undergo a multitude of changes, and one of the most crucial systems affected is the digestive system. The aging digestive system demands special considerations and care to maintain overall health and well-being. Here, we delve into the intricacies of this vital bodily function and explore the measures necessary for its optimal functioning as we age.

- Slowing Metabolism: With age, our metabolism gradually slows down. This means that the body processes food at a slower rate, leading to a decreased calorie requirement. It is crucial to adapt one's diet accordingly to avoid weight gain. Incorporating more nutrient-dense foods and reducing empty calories from sugars and fats can help maintain a healthy weight.

- **Digestive Enzyme Production:** The production of digestive enzymes, such as amylase and lipase, tends to decline with age. As a result, older adults may have difficulty breaking down certain foods, leading to discomfort and nutrient malabsorption. To counteract this, consider enzyme supplements or consuming foods that are easier to digest, such as yogurt or cooked vegetables.

- **Hydration:** Aging can sometimes lead to reduced sensation of thirst, which may result in inadequate fluid intake. Dehydration can have severe consequences on digestion, making it crucial for older individuals to drink sufficient water throughout the day. Herbal teas, broths, and water-rich fruits like watermelon can also contribute to hydration.

- **Fiber Intake:** Maintaining regularity in bowel movements becomes increasingly important as the digestive system ages. Fiber-rich foods, including whole grains, fruits, and vegetables, are essential for preventing constipation and promoting a healthy gut. Adequate fiber intake can also help lower the risk of digestive disorders like diverticulosis.

- Probiotics: The balance of beneficial bacteria in the gut can be disrupted as we age. This can result in gastrointestinal issues and a weakened immune system. Probiotic-rich foods like yogurt, kefir, and fermented vegetables can help restore this balance, improving digestion and overall health.

- Medication Interactions: Many older adults take multiple medications, some of which may have adverse effects on digestion. It's essential to consult with a healthcare professional to understand how medications may impact your digestive system and whether dietary adjustments or additional medications may be necessary to counteract these effects.

- **Chewing and Mealtime Habits:** Chewing becomes even more critical as we age since it aids in breaking down food for digestion. Older adults may benefit from taking their time to chew food thoroughly and avoid rushing meals. Smaller, more frequent meals can also be easier to digest than large, heavy ones.

- **Food Sensitivities:** Age-related changes in the digestive tract can lead to the development of food sensitivities or intolerances. Pay attention to how your body reacts to certain foods, and if you suspect sensitivities, consider keeping a food diary or consulting a healthcare professional for guidance.

- **Regular Check-ups:** Aging individuals should maintain regular check-ups with healthcare providers, including gastroenterologists, to monitor the health of their digestive system. Screening for conditions like colorectal cancer and managing chronic digestive conditions is essential for early detection and effective management.

The aging digestive system requires special attention and care to ensure optimal health and well-being. By adjusting dietary habits, staying hydrated, and seeking medical guidance when necessary, individuals can navigate the challenges of an aging digestive system while maintaining their overall quality of life.

Chapter 2: Weight Loss Diet Basics

The Weight Loss Diet Principles

Foods to Embrace

Embracing a wholesome and nourishing diet is essential for promoting good health and well-being. The choices we make in our daily meals can have a profound impact on our energy levels, longevity, and overall quality of life. Below, we explore a diverse array of foods that offer a treasure trove of health benefits, each contributing in its own unique way to a balanced and vibrant lifestyle.

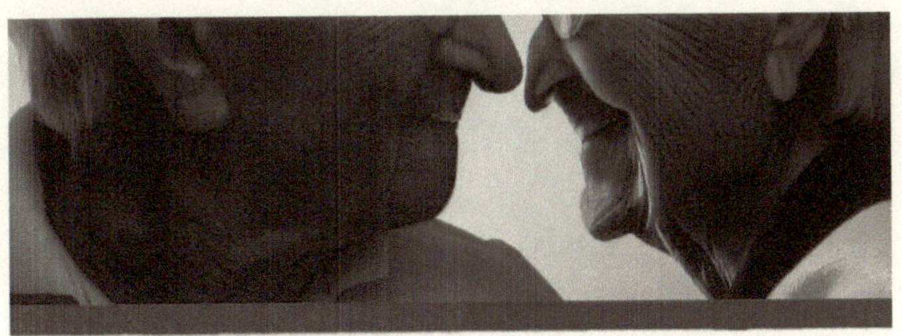

HEALTHY SENIOR DIET

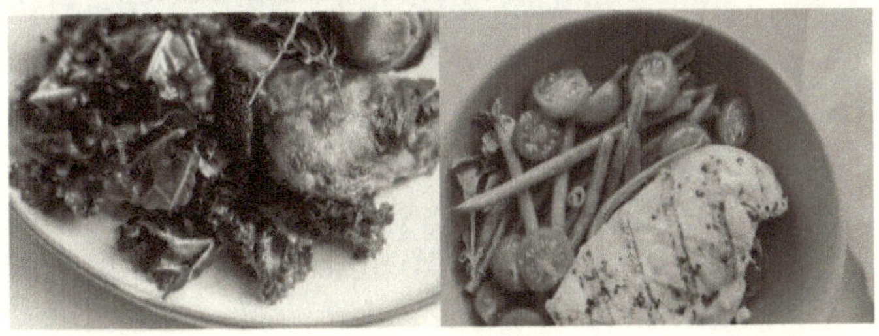

•Leafy Greens: Dark, leafy greens such as spinach, kale, and Swiss chard are packed with vitamins, minerals, and antioxidants. They promote heart health, bolster the immune system, and support healthy skin.

- Berries: Blueberries, strawberries, and raspberries are rich in antioxidants, known to combat oxidative stress and reduce the risk of chronic diseases. They're also low in calories and high in fiber.

- **Fatty Fish:** Salmon, mackerel, and sardines are teeming with omega-3 fatty acids, which are excellent for heart health and may reduce the risk of cognitive decline.
- **Nuts and Seeds:** Such as almonds, walnuts, flaxseeds, and chia seeds provide healthy fats, protein, and fiber. They're ideal for snacking and can help control appetite.
- **Whole Grains:** Oats, quinoa, and brown rice are fiber-rich options that stabilize blood sugar levels and keep you feeling full for longer. This is also a source of essential nutrients.
- **Legumes:** Lentils, chickpeas, and black beans are plant-based protein powerhouses. They're excellent for vegetarians and vegans and help regulate blood sugar.
- **Yogurt and Fermented Foods:** These are rich in probiotics that support gut

health and boost the immune system. Look for unsweetened options to minimize added sugars.

- Cruciferous Vegetables: Broccoli, cauliflower, and Brussels sprouts contain compounds that may reduce the risk of cancer and promote detoxification in the body.
- Tomatoes: Tomatoes are a source of lycopene, an antioxidant that may lower the risk of certain cancers. They're also a versatile ingredient in various dishes.
- Herbs and Spices: Turmeric, ginger, and garlic have potent anti-inflammatory properties. They can be added to dishes or consumed as teas for their health benefits.
- Lean Proteins: Skinless poultry, lean cuts of beef, and tofu are sources of high-quality protein that aid in muscle repair and immune function.
- Avocado: Avocado is a nutrient-dense fruit loaded with healthy fats and fiber. It's great for heart health and

can be used in salads, sandwiches, or as a topping.

- **Eggs:** Eggs are a fantastic source of protein and essential nutrients like choline, which supports brain health. These are also versatile and can be prepared in various ways.
- **Dark Chocolate:** In moderation, dark chocolate (with a high cocoa content) is rich in antioxidants and may improve heart health. It's a delightful treat for occasional indulgence.
- **Green Tea:** Green tea is known for its antioxidant properties and potential benefits for weight management and cognitive function.

Remember that a balanced diet is about variety and moderation. Embrace these foods as part of a well-rounded meal plan, and be mindful of portion sizes. Prioritize whole, unprocessed foods, and stay hydrated with plenty of water. A diet that incorporates these foods can be a powerful step toward a healthier, more vibrant life.

Foods to Avoid

Maintaining good health and well-being is a priority for many, and one of the most influential factors in achieving this is our diet. What we eat directly impacts our energy levels, weight, mood, and overall longevity. While there's no one-size-fits-all approach to nutrition, there are certain foods that are universally recognized as needing limitation or avoidance. Here, we explore these dietary culprits and why they should be consumed in moderation or, in some cases, not at all.

1. Sugary Beverages:

Sugary drinks, such as soda, fruit juices, and energy drinks, are loaded with empty calories. This can contribute to weight gain, increase the risk of type 2 diabetes, and harm dental health. You can opt for water, herbal tea, or unsweetened beverages instead.

2. Processed Meats:

Processed meats like hot dogs, bacon, and deli meats are often high in saturated fats, sodium, and preservatives. Regular consumption has been linked to an increased risk of heart disease and certain cancers.Lean, unprocessed meats or plant-based alternatives can be chosen.

3. Trans Fats:

Trans fats, often found in partially hydrogenated oils, are known to raise bad cholesterol (LDL) levels and lower good cholesterol (HDL). They are commonly found in fast food, fried snacks, and some baked goods. Always check food labels and avoid products with trans fats.

4. Highly Processed Foods:

Foods high in artificial additives, preservatives, and refined ingredients offer little nutritional value and may contribute to overeating. Instead, focus on whole, minimally processed foods like, vegetables, and whole grains.

5. Excessive Salt (Sodium):

High sodium intake can lead to hypertension and increase the risk of stroke, heart disease, and kidney problems. Reduce salt by avoiding heavily processed foods, using herbs and spices for flavor, and checking food labels for sodium content.

6. Added Sugars:

Excessive sugar consumption can lead to obesity, type 2 diabetes, and dental issues. Limit sugary snacks, cereals, and desserts, and be cautious of hidden sugars in sauces and condiments.

7. White Bread and Refined Grains:

Refined grains like white bread lack the fiber and nutrients found in whole grains. They can cause rapid spikes in blood sugar levels. You can opt for whole grain options like whole wheat bread, brown rice, and quinoa.

8. Alcohol in Excess:

While moderate alcohol consumption may have some health benefits, excessive drinking can lead to liver damage, addiction, and a range of health issues. Be mindful of your alcohol intake and drink responsibly.

9. Saturated Fats:

Saturated fats, often found in red meat, full-fat dairy, and fried foods, can raise cholesterol levels and increase the risk of heart disease. Choose lean protein sources and use healthier cooking oils.

10. Artificial Sweeteners:

Artificial sweeteners, found in many diet sodas and sugar-free products, may not be as benign as once thought. Some studies suggest they could have negative effects on metabolism and appetite regulation. Moderation is key.

A very balanced and nutritious diet is essential for good health. While these foods should be limited or avoided, remember that occasional indulgence is okay. The key is to make informed choices, prioritize whole foods, and maintain a sustainable, balanced approach to eating. Consult with a healthcare professional or registered dietitian for personalized guidance on your dietary needs and goals.

Incorporating Superfoods into Your Diet

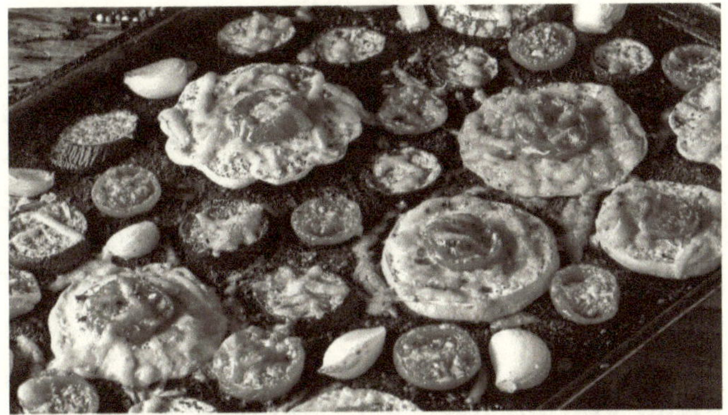

In today's fast-paced world, the maintaining of a healthy diet can be a challenge. However, the concept of "superfoods" has gained significant attention in recent years, offering a promising solution to enhance our overall well-being. These nutrient-packed, natural wonders have the potential to revolutionize your diet and pave the way to a healthier, more vibrant you. In this comprehensive guide, we delve into the fascinating world of superfoods and provide actionable tips on how to seamlessly incorporate them into your daily meals.

Understanding Superfoods:

Superfoods are not mythical potions; they are real, whole foods that are packed with an abundance of essential nutrients, antioxidants, and health-boosting compounds. These extraordinary edibles have been shown to reduce the risk of chronic diseases, support weight management, and boost overall vitality. From vibrant berries to nutrient-dense leafy greens, superfoods offer a spectrum of flavors and textures to explore.

Selecting Your Superfoods:

- **Berries Galore:** Start with a colorful assortment of berries – blueberries, strawberries, raspberries, and blackberries. These tiny titans are brimming with antioxidants, vitamins, and fiber that help combat oxidative stress and support heart health.

- **Leafy Greens:** Incorporate leafy greens like kale, spinach, and Swiss chard into your salads and smoothies. Rich in vitamins A, C, and K, these greens bolster your immune system and promote bone health.
- **Omega-3 Power:** Incorporate fatty fish such as salmon, mackerel, and sardines into your diet for a dose of omega-3 fatty acids. These healthy fats are renowned for their brain-boosting and heart-protective benefits.
- **Ancient Grains:** Replace refined grains with ancient grains like quinoa, farro, and amaranth. These whole grains are packed with fiber and essential amino acids, promoting sustained energy and digestive health.
- **Cruciferous Champions:** Broccoli, cauliflower, and Brussels sprouts are cruciferous vegetables that are rich in

cancer-fighting compounds and offer a wealth of vitamins and minerals.

Incorporating Superfoods:

- Smoothie Sensation: Blend a handful of spinach or kale with berries, a banana, Greek yogurt, and a sprinkle of chia seeds for a nutrient-packed breakfast on the go.
- Salad Supercharge: Add diced avocado, walnuts, and pomegranate seeds to your salads to enhance flavor and boost nutrition.
- Superfood Bowls: Create nourishing bowls with a base of quinoa or brown rice, topped with grilled salmon, steamed broccoli, and a drizzle of olive oil.
- Snack Smart: Swap processed snacks with a small handful of almonds or walnuts and a side of fresh fruit for a satisfying and healthy midday pick-me-up.
- Herb and Spice Magic: Experiment with herbs and spices like turmeric,

ginger, and cinnamon in your cooking. These flavor enhancers also offer anti-inflammatory properties.

Incorporating superfoods into your diet is a journey toward a healthier, more vibrant life. By harnessing the power of nutrient-dense, natural ingredients, you can take proactive steps to boost your well-being and reduce the risk of chronic illnesses. Start small, experiment with flavors, and gradually transform your daily meals into a symphony of superfood goodness. Remember, this is not just about eating well; it's about living well. Embrace the superfoods, and let them be your allies on the path to optimal health and vitality.

Chapter 3: Meal Planning for Seniors

Weekly Meal Planning Guide

Sample Weight Loss Diet Meal Plans

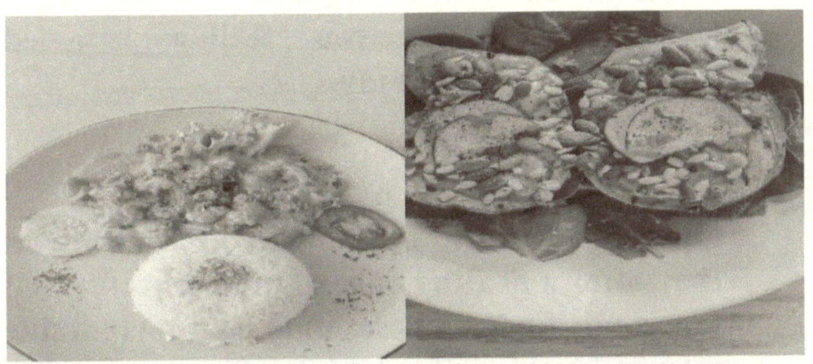

In a world saturated with fad diets promising rapid weight loss, the Weight Loss Diet stands as a beacon of sustainable, long-term health. Rooted in the principle of maintaining stable insulin levels, this approach to eating isn't just about shedding pounds; it's about fostering overall wellness. Let's delve into a detailed sample meal plan

that exemplifies the Weight Loss Diet's philosophy.

Breakfast:

Start your day with a balanced blend of protein, healthy fats, and complex carbohydrates. A spinach and feta omelet with whole-grain toast and a side of avocado provides a nutrient-packed foundation. This combination helps regulate blood sugar levels and keeps you feeling satisfied throughout the morning.

Morning Snack:

Opt for a handful of almonds or walnuts, as they offer a healthy dose of monounsaturated fats and fiber. These nuts support stable insulin levels while staving off mid-morning hunger pangs.

Lunch:

A colorful salad featuring lean protein like grilled chicken or chickpeas, along with a variety of veggies, will keep you energized.

Top it off with a vinaigrette made from olive oil and balsamic vinegar to maintain healthy blood sugar levels.

Afternoon Snack:

Greek yogurt with berries and a sprinkle of cinnamon is both delicious and nutritious. The yogurt provides protein, while the berries offer antioxidants and fiber, and cinnamon may help regulate blood sugar.

Dinner:

For dinner, a serving of wild-caught salmon or tofu, accompanied by steamed broccoli and quinoa, makes for a balanced, low-GI (glycemic index) meal. The Omega-3 fatty acids in salmon contribute to insulin sensitivity, while quinoa provides complex carbohydrates without the blood sugar spikes.

Evening Snack (optional):

If you need a little something before bed, consider a small portion of cottage cheese with a drizzle of honey. This combines protein and a touch of natural sweetness, promoting stable blood sugar even during sleep.

Hydration:

Throughout the day, remember to stay well-hydrated with water or herbal teas. Proper hydration supports metabolic function and can aid in appetite control.

Key Principles of the Golo Diet:

- Balanced Macronutrients: Each meal includes a mix of protein, healthy fats, and complex carbohydrates to stabilize blood sugar levels and prevent spikes.
- Whole Foods: Emphasis is placed on unprocessed, whole foods, rich in nutrients, and low in refined sugars and artificial additives.
- Portion Control: Mindful portion sizes are encouraged to prevent overeating and maintain steady insulin levels.

- **Regular Meals and Snacks:** Consistent eating intervals help avoid blood sugar crashes and curb unhealthy cravings.
- **Sustainable Lifestyle:** The Golo Diet is not a quick fix but a sustainable approach to healthy eating and living, promoting long-term weight management and overall well-being.
- **Supplement Support:** Some individuals may choose to complement their diet with the Golo Release supplement, which contains natural ingredients aimed at supporting metabolic health.

By adhering to the Weight Loss Diet's core principles and adopting a meal plan like the one described above, you're not only taking steps towards weight management but also nurturing your body's overall health and vitality. Remember, it's not just about losing weight; it's about embracing a lifestyle that promotes well-being for years to come.

Cooking Tips for Seniors

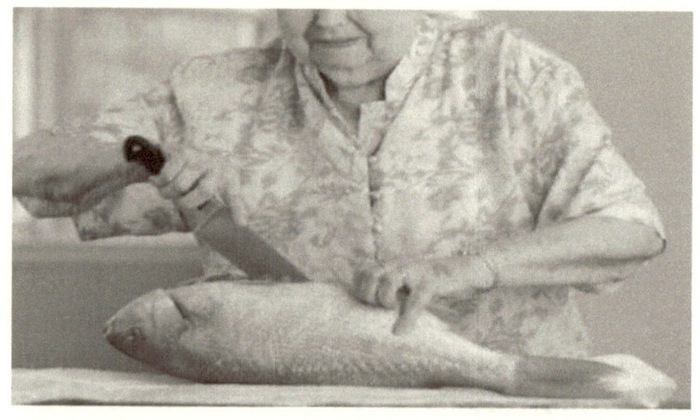

Cooking is a fundamental life skill, and as we age, it becomes even more critical for maintaining independence and overall well-being. Seniors often face unique challenges in the kitchen, from limited mobility to dietary restrictions. However, with the right guidance and a few adjustments, seniors can continue to enjoy the pleasures of cooking while ensuring safety and nutrition. Here are some valuable cooking tips tailored to seniors:

- **Plan Your Meals:** Get started by planning your meals for the week. This not only helps you stay organized but also ensures a balanced diet.

Include a variety of colorful fruits and vegetables, lean proteins, and whole grains in your plan.

- Preparation is Key: Prepping ingredients in advance can save you time and effort. Consider chopping vegetables, portioning meats, and measuring ingredients before you start cooking.
- Invest in Kitchen Aids: Modern kitchen gadgets can be a real game-changer for seniors. Electric can openers, jar openers, and food processors can make tasks easier and reduce the strain on your hands and wrists.
- Opt for Convenience: Frozen vegetables and pre-cut fruits can be convenient options without sacrificing nutrition. This shows they have a longer shelf life and require minimal preparation.
- Use Smaller Cookware: Smaller pots and pans are easier to handle and clean. Consider non-stick cookware, which reduces the need for excessive

oils and makes cooking and cleaning a breeze.

- **Master One-Pot Dishes:** Casseroles, stir-fries, and one-pot meals are not only delicious but also simplify cooking and reduce the number of dishes to clean.
- **Slow Cookers and Instant Pots:** These appliances are seniors' best friends. They allow you to prepare flavorful, nutritious meals with minimal effort. Just set it and forget it!
- **Mindful Seasoning:** Reduce sodium intake by using herbs, spices, and citrus to flavor your dishes. Experiment with flavors to make your meals exciting.
- **Stay Hydrated:** Don't forget to drink water while you cook. Dehydration can lead to fatigue and confusion. Try to keep a glass or a bottle of water nearby.
- **Practice Safety:** Always prioritize safety in the kitchen. Install anti-slip mats, use oven mitts, and be cautious around hot surfaces. If you have

mobility issues, consider using a sturdy stool or chair for support.

- Ask for Help: Don't hesitate to seek assistance from family members, friends, or caregivers when needed. Cooking can be a social activity, and sharing the kitchen can be enjoyable.
- Maintain a Clean Kitchen: Keep your kitchen clean and clutter-free. Regularly check the expiry dates of food items to ensure you're using fresh ingredients.
- Portion Control: Seniors often have different dietary needs. Pay attention to portion sizes to avoid overeating and to ensure you get the right nutrients.
- Explore New Recipes: Cooking can be a creative outlet. Try out new recipes to keep things interesting and exciting in the kitchen.
- Stay Informed: Keep up to date with the latest nutrition guidelines and health recommendations. Make sure you consult with a healthcare

professional or dietitian for personalized advice.

Cooking is not just about sustenance; it's an expression of independence and creativity. By following these cooking tips, seniors can continue to enjoy delicious and nutritious meals while staying safe and self-sufficient in the kitchen.

Dining Out the Weight Loss Way

Imagine a dining experience that transcends mere sustenance and elevates your senses to new heights. This is the essence of dining out the Weight loss way, a culinary journey that promises to be unforgettable. In this gastronomic adventure, we'll explore the key elements that define this unique approach to dining, offering a tantalizing glimpse into a world where food becomes art.

- **The Weight Loss Philosophy:** At the heart of the Weight Loss way lies a deep appreciation for food as a form of art, a means of connection, and a source of nourishment. This philosophy emphasizes the importance of savoring every bite, celebrating ingredients, and relishing the entire dining experience.

- **Mindful Selection:** Weight Loss dining begins with a thoughtful selection of the restaurant. Seek out establishments that prioritize sustainable sourcing, local ingredients, and a commitment to culinary innovation. Weight Loss enthusiasts are discerning patrons who value quality over quantity.

- **Exploration through the Menu:** Once seated, the Weight Loss diner embarks on a culinary journey through the menu. Rather than hastily choosing familiar dishes, they take time to study the offerings, considering flavors, textures, and the stories behind each creation. This exploration is not rushed; it's a ritual of anticipation.

- **Engaging with the Chef:** The Weight Loss way often involves interacting with the chef or kitchen staff. This connection allows for a personalized experience, where the chef can craft dishes that suit your preferences, dietary needs, and even surprise you with culinary delights.

- **Appreciation of Presentation:** In Weight Loss dining, presentation is as important as taste. Each dish is a work of art, carefully arranged on the plate to engage your visual senses. The interplay of colors, shapes, and textures adds an extra layer of excitement to the meal.
- **Savoring Every Bite:** Weight Loss diners savor each bite, paying attention to the various flavors and sensations that dance on their palate. They appreciate the complex symphony of tastes that a well-crafted dish can offer.
- **Wine Pairing:** A Weight Loss dining experience often includes wine pairing. A skilled sommelier can enhance the flavors of each dish with a perfectly chosen wine, elevating the overall experience.

- **Sharing and Conversation:** Dining out the Weight Loss way is not a solitary endeavor. It's a social experience meant to be shared with friends or loved ones. Engaging conversation and shared appreciation for the food enhance the meal.

- **Dessert as a Grand Finale:** Dessert is not an afterthought; it's the grand finale of the Weight Loss dining experience. A well-crafted dessert can be a culmination of flavors, textures, and creativity, leaving a lasting impression.

- **Gratitude:** The Weight Loss way is not just about indulgence; it's about gratitude. Express appreciation to the chef and staff for their dedication to creating a memorable dining experience.

Dining out the Weight Loss way is a celebration of the culinary arts, a sensory journey that engages the mind, heart, and palate. It's a reminder that food is not just sustenance but a means of experiencing the world's diversity, creativity, and beauty. So, the next time you dine out, consider adopting the Weight Loss philosophy and embark on a culinary adventure that will leave you with memories to savor for a lifetime.

Chapter 4: Senior-Friendly Recipes

Breakfast Delights

- Savory **Soups and Stews**

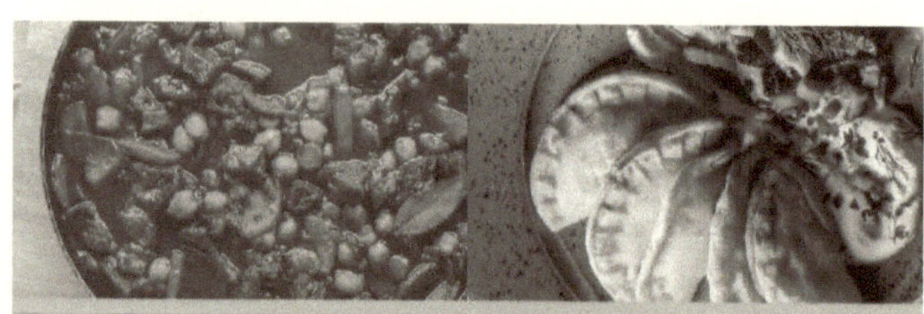

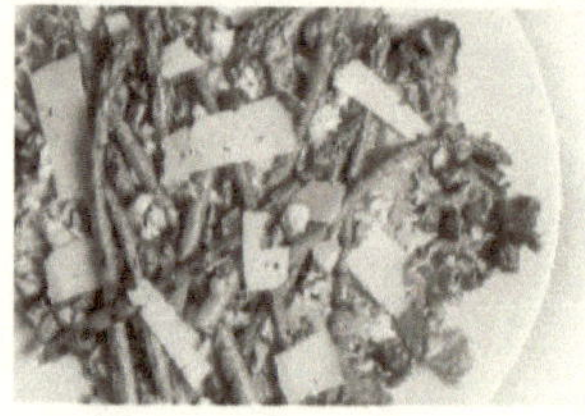

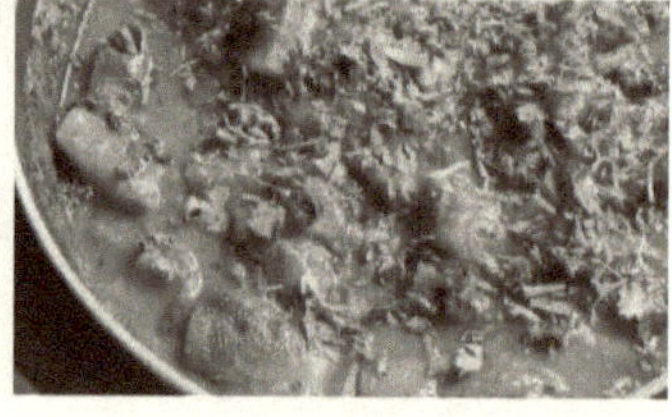

As we gracefully age, the importance of a balanced and nourishing diet becomes ever more significant. Among the various culinary delights that offer both taste and nutrition, savory soups and stews stand as timeless favorites. These wholesome dishes not only warm the soul but also provide seniors with a plethora of health benefits.

- **Nutrient-Rich Goodness:** Savory soups and stews are culinary treasures packed with essential nutrients. They often feature a medley of vegetables, lean proteins, and legumes, ensuring a well-rounded meal in a single bowl. The slow simmering process allows for the release of vitamins and minerals, making these dishes a powerhouse of nutrition.
- **Gentle on Digestion:** One of the advantages of soups and stews for seniors is their gentle impact on digestion. The slow cooking process breaks down ingredients, making them easier to chew and digest. This is particularly beneficial for individuals with dental issues or those experiencing age-related digestive challenges.

- **Hydration Heroes:** Staying adequately hydrated is crucial for seniors, and soups and stews help in this regard. Their high water content not only satisfies thirst but also contributes to overall hydration. This is especially important as the sensation of thirst often diminishes with age.
- **Flavorful Variety:** The world of savory soups and stews is virtually limitless, offering a wide array of flavors and cultural influences. From hearty beef stew to fragrant vegetable broth and exotic international offerings like Thai Tom Yum soup, there's something to tantalize every senior's taste buds.
- **Managing Sodium:** Seniors often need to monitor their sodium intake. Homemade soups and stews give them control over the salt content, allowing for a heart-healthy option. Low-sodium broths and herbs and spices can be used to enhance flavor without compromising on health.

- **Bone Health:** Many seniors are concerned about bone health. The inclusion of bone-in cuts of meat in stews and the use of bone broth as a base provide a natural source of calcium and other minerals essential for maintaining strong bones.
- **Weight Management:** Soups and stews can be tailored to suit various dietary needs, including those aiming for weight management. By choosing lean proteins and incorporating a variety of vegetables, seniors can enjoy a filling meal with fewer calories.
- **Social and Emotional Benefits:** Sharing a bowl of soup or stew with loved ones can be a heartwarming experience. These dishes encourage social interaction and foster a sense of connection, combating feelings of loneliness and isolation that some seniors may face.
- **Easy Preparation:** For seniors who prefer simplicity in the kitchen, soups and stews are a dream come true. They can be prepared in advance,

- **frozen for later use, or made in large batches to provide nourishment for days to come.**

Savory soups and stews are a culinary embrace for seniors. They offer a delightful blend of flavor and nutrition, catering to the unique dietary needs of older individuals. Whether enjoyed for their comfort, ease of preparation, or the nutritional benefits they bring, these dishes remain a cherished part of a well-rounded senior diet.

- **Healthy Salads and Sides**

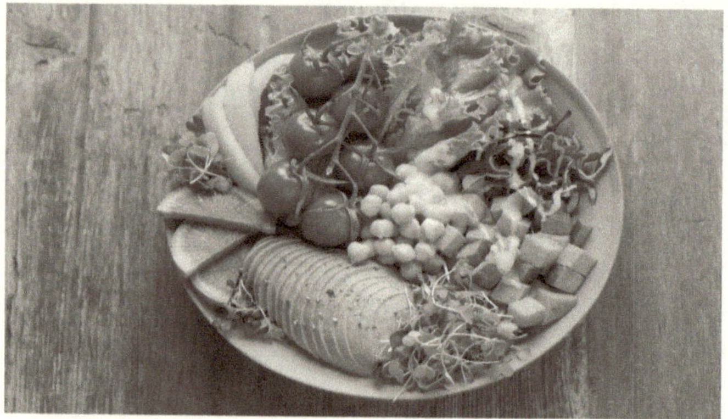

As we age, maintaining a well balanced and nutritious diet becomes increasingly important for our overall health and well-being. One of the most delightful and beneficial ways to achieve this is through a diverse selection of healthy salads and sides. These dishes not only offer a burst of flavors but also provide seniors with essential nutrients, fiber, and hydration. Here, we explore some delectable options that are tailored to the unique nutritional needs of seniors.

1. Leafy Green Wonders

Seniors can benefit greatly from leafy greens like spinach, kale, and arugula. These greens are rich in vitamins K, A, and C, which support bone health and boost the immune system. Toss them with a light vinaigrette and top with roasted nuts or seeds for added texture and healthy fats.

2. Protein-Packed Quinoa Salad

Quinoa is a complete protein source, making it an ideal addition to senior diets. Combine cooked quinoa with colorful bell peppers, cucumber, and cherry tomatoes for a vibrant and protein-rich salad. Add a sprinkle of feta cheese or chickpeas for extra protein and flavor.

3. Fiber-Rich Fruit Salad

Seniors should aim to include plenty of fiber in their diet to aid digestion. Create a refreshing fruit salad with a mix of berries, apples, and citrus fruits. These fruits are not only high in fiber but also provide a dose of antioxidants and vitamins.

4. Creamy Avocado Delight

Avocados are a fantastic source of healthy fats and potassium. Create a creamy avocado salad by mashing ripe avocados and mixing them with diced tomatoes, red onion, and a squeeze of lime juice. This is not only nutritious but also easy to eat for seniors with dental concerns.

5. Roasted Vegetable Medley

Roasting vegetables like carrots, sweet potatoes, and broccoli brings out their natural sweetness and enhances their flavor. These veggies are rich in vitamins and antioxidants, making them a superb side dish for seniors. A touch of olive oil, garlic, and herbs can elevate the taste.

6. Greek Tzatziki Cucumber Salad

Tzatziki salad is a cooling and delicious option, particularly during hot weather. Combine diced cucumbers with Greek yogurt, garlic, dill, and a splash of lemon juice. It's a great source of probiotics, calcium, and hydration.

7. Nutrient-Packed Quinoa Stuffed Peppers

Hollowed-out bell peppers make a perfect vessel for stuffing with a mixture of cooked quinoa, lean ground turkey or tofu, and an array of finely chopped vegetables. This dish is not only visually appealing but also rich in protein, fiber, and vitamins.

8. Light and Lively Coleslaw

Create a healthier version of coleslaw by using Greek yogurt or a light dressing instead of mayonnaise. Shredded cabbage and carrots provide vitamins and fiber while remaining easy to chew. Incorporate raisins or diced apples for a touch of natural sweetness.

9. Hummus and Veggie Platter

A colorful platter of sliced bell peppers, cherry tomatoes, cucumber, and baby carrots served with a side of hummus is a delightful and nutritious snack or side dish. Hummus is a very good source of plant-based protein and fiber.

10. Hydrating Watermelon Salad

In warm weather, nothing beats the refreshing taste of watermelon. Combine diced watermelon with feta cheese, mint leaves, and a drizzle of balsamic glaze for a hydrating and sweet-savory salad.

These healthy salads and sides not only cater to the nutritional needs of seniors but also offer a variety of tastes and textures to keep mealtimes enjoyable. Customizing these dishes to personal preferences and dietary restrictions ensures thats seniors can savor every bite while supporting their health and vitality.

Main Course Meals

As we journey through life, our dietary needs evolve, and this is especially true for seniors. Main course meals for this demographic require careful consideration, not only for their nutritional requirements but also to ensure they savor each bite. Let's explore a range of main course options designed to cater to the unique needs and tastes of seniors.

- Salmon with Lemon-Dill Sauce: This dish offers a trifecta of benefits. The salmon provides essential omega-3 fatty acids for heart and brain health. The zesty lemon-dill sauce adds a burst of flavor while being gentle on the palate. Accompanied by steamed vegetables, this meal is a nutritious masterpiece.

- Chicken and Vegetable Stir-Fry: Seniors need protein to maintain muscle mass, and this dish delivers. Tender pieces of chicken, sautéed with an array of colorful vegetables, not only provide protein but also a wealth of vitamins and antioxidants. The stir-fry's gentle spices make it suitable for sensitive taste buds.
- Mushroom Risotto: Creamy, comforting, and easy to digest, mushroom risotto is a perfect choice for seniors. The rice provides sustenance, while the earthy mushrooms offer depth of flavor. A dash of Parmesan cheese adds a touch of luxury to this classic Italian dish.
- Baked Sweet Potato with Turkey: Sweet potatoes are a nutritional powerhouse, rich in fiber and vitamins. Topped with lean ground turkey, seasoned with herbs and spices, this dish is both satisfying and low in saturated fats. It's a superb

option for seniors watching their cholesterol.

- **Vegetable Lasagna:** A vegetarian delight, vegetable lasagna combines layers of pasta with a medley of roasted vegetables and a velvety béchamel sauce. It's a comforting, easy-to-chew alternative for seniors who prefer plant-based options.
- **Beef Stew:** Slow-cooked beef stew is a timeless favorite. Tender chunks of beef, carrots, potatoes, and onions simmered in a flavorful broth create a hearty meal. The stew's gentle cooking process ensures that meat is tender and easily digestible.
- **Quinoa and Black Bean Bowl:** Quinoa is a superfood that packs protein and fiber, making it an ideal choice for seniors. Combined with black beans, colorful bell peppers, and a zesty lime dressing, this dish is a nutritional powerhouse with a southwestern twist.
- **Spinach and Cheese Stuffed Chicken Breast:** This dish combines lean chicken breast with a filling of spinach

and low-fat cheese. Baked to perfection, it's not only high in protein but also a good source of calcium and iron, essential for senior bone health.

- Eggplant Parmesan: Layers of breaded and baked eggplant slices, smothered in marinara sauce and melted cheese, create a comforting Italian classic. It's a wonderful choice for seniors who appreciate the flavors of traditional comfort food.
- Salad Niçoise: A refreshing option for warmer days, Salad Niçoise features tuna, boiled eggs, olives, and fresh vegetables over a bed of crisp lettuce. Drizzled with a vinaigrette, it's a light yet satisfying main course option.

Remember, presentation and portion size play a significant role in making these meals appealing to seniors. Smaller, well-plated servings can enhance the dining experience. Additionally, it's crucial to consider any dietary restrictions or allergies individual seniors may have.

In crafting main course meals for seniors, the goal is to nourish not only their bodies but also their spirits. A thoughtful and varied menu that prioritizes taste, texture, and nutrition can transform mealtimes into enjoyable and fulfilling moments.

Snacks and Treats

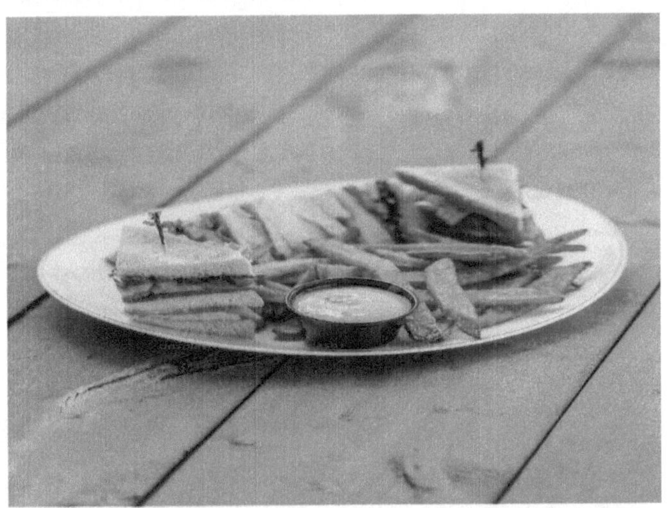

As we journey through life, our tastes and dietary needs evolve, and this rings especially true for seniors. Snacks and treats for our beloved older generation aren't just about satisfying hunger; they're a bridge to nostalgia, a source of comfort, and a means of promoting overall well-being. Let's explore the world of snacks and treats designed with seniors in mind.

- **Nutrition Meets Delight:** Senior snacks should strike a balance between nutrition and indulgence. Consider options like whole-grain crackers with low-fat cheese or yogurt-covered almonds. These snacks provide essential nutrients while pleasing the taste buds.
- **Fruitful Delights:** Fresh fruits, whether in their natural form or dried, are a treasure trove of vitamins, fiber, and natural sweetness. Seniors can enjoy a medley of apple slices with a sprinkle of cinnamon or apricots as a delicious and healthy snack.
- **Nostalgic Joy:** Remind seniors of simpler times with classic treats like oatmeal cookies or rice pudding. These timeless favorites evoke cherished

memories and offer comfort like no other.

- **Savory Satisfaction:** Seniors may prefer savory over sweet. Opt for options like air-popped popcorn with a dash of herbs or vegetable sticks with hummus. These snacks are not only tasty but also easy on the waistline.
- **Hydration Helpers:** Dehydration can be a concern for seniors. Encourage them to snack on juicy watermelon chunks or cucumber slices, both of which provide hydration along with a refreshing taste.
- **Mini-Meals:** Sometimes, seniors may prefer smaller, more frequent snacks rather than traditional meals. Create mini-meals with a variety of items like whole-grain crackers, lean protein slices, and a selection of colorful, crunchy veggies.
- **Texture Matters:** Dental health can be a concern for older individuals. Choose snacks that are easy to chew, like soft granola bars, ripe bananas, or smoothies packed with nutrients.

- **Spice It Up:** For those who enjoy a bit of zest, consider adding a dash of spice. Seniors can explore the world of flavored nuts or baked sweet potato fries with a sprinkle of paprika for a flavorful kick.
- **Tea Time:** A warm cup of herbal tea can be a soothing snack option. Herbal teas like chamomile or peppermint not only taste delightful but can also aid digestion and promote relaxation.
- **Customize to Preferences:** Every senior has unique tastes and dietary requirements. Engage with them to discover their favorites and tailor snacks accordingly. This personal touch can make all the difference you want.

Snacks and treats for seniors are a gateway to both physical nourishment and emotional well-being. These small delights have the power to evoke cherished memories, nourish the body, and bring comfort to the soul. It's a thoughtful way to show appreciation and care for our seniors, ensuring their twilight years are filled with flavor, joy, and love.

Desserts for a Sweet Treat

In the tapestry of life, the golden years are the threads that weave stories of wisdom, love, and cherished memories. For our beloved seniors, every moment deserves to be celebrated, and what better way to bring joy and sweetness into their lives than with a delectable array of desserts? Desserts are not just confections; they are expressions of love, nostalgia, and the simple pleasure of savoring life's sweetness.

Picture a sunny afternoon, with a gentle breeze rustling through the leaves, as seniors gather around a beautifully set table adorned with an enticing assortment of desserts. The scene is set for a delightful treat that goes beyond the sugary surface to evoke emotions, trigger memories, and create lasting bonds.

Let's embark on a journey through the world of desserts tailor-made for our cherished seniors:

- Classic Apple Pie: A slice of warm apple pie, with its flaky crust and aromatic cinnamon-spiced apples, is like a hug from grandma. Served with a dollop of vanilla ice cream, it's a timeless favorite that transports taste buds to the heart of nostalgia.
- Creamy Rice Pudding: Creamy, comforting, and crowned with a sprinkle of cinnamon, rice pudding is a cozy dessert that whispers of home. It's a humble delight that soothes the soul with each spoonful.
- Decadent Chocolate Mousse: Dark chocolate mousse, with its velvety texture and rich cocoa flavor, is a testament to the finer things in life. Topped with a garnish of fresh berries, it's a treat that delights both the eyes and the palate.
- Lemon Bars: The zesty tang of lemon bars awakens the senses and offers a

burst of sunshine. The sweet and tart flavors dance harmoniously on the taste buds, leaving behind a sense of zest for life.

- **Delicate Tea Cakes:** Delicate tea cakes, adorned with powdered sugar and served with a side of tea or coffee, create a perfect moment of calm. These bite-sized wonders are an invitation to savor the present.
- **Fresh Fruit Salad:** A rainbow of fresh fruits, carefully diced and artfully arranged, not only satisfies the sweet tooth but also nourishes the body and soul. It's a celebration of nature's bounty.
- **Almond Biscotti:** Crisp, twice-baked almond biscotti is a delightful companion to a cup of hot coffee. Its subtle nuttiness and satisfying crunch make it a wonderful treat for seniors to savor.
- **Cherry Cheesecake:** A velvety cheesecake crowned with ruby-red cherries is a symphony of flavors and

textures. This is a dessert that embodies elegance and indulgence.

- Banana Bread: Moist and fragrant, banana bread is a slice of home-baked comfort. Its subtle sweetness and familiar aroma evoke cherished memories of kitchens filled with laughter.
- Assorted Petit Fours: A platter of petit fours offers a bite-sized journey through a world of flavors. From mini eclairs to dainty macarons, these tiny treasures are a delightful surprise with each nibble.

Desserts are not just about satisfying cravings; they're about creating moments of connection and delight. They're a gesture of love and appreciation for the wisdom and experiences our seniors have shared with us. So, let's serve up these sweet treasures and create memories as rich and timeless as the flavors themselves, for our beloved seniors deserve nothing less.

Chapter 5: Special Health Considerations

Managing Diabetes and Blood Sugar

Heart Health and Hypertension

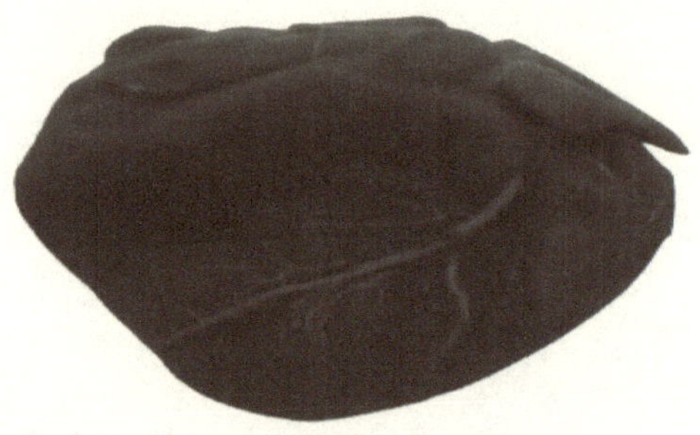

Maintaining heart health is a crucial aspect of overall well-being, especially for seniors. As we age, our bodies undergo various changes, and the cardiovascular system is no exception. Heart-related issues become more prevalent, with hypertension, or high blood pressure, emerging as a common concern. This comprehensive guide explores the intricacies of heart health and hypertension in seniors, offering valuable insights and recommendations to lead a heart-healthy life.

Understanding the Aging Heart

As we age, our heart undergoes natural changes that can impact its efficiency. Key changes include a decrease in the heart's ability to pump blood effectively, a stiffening of arteries, and a potential increase in blood pressure. Seniors should be aware of these changes to better manage their heart health.

The Impact of Hypertension

Hypertension, often referred to as the "silent killer," is a leading risk factor for heart disease, stroke, and other cardiovascular issues. Seniors are particularly susceptible to hypertension due to age-related changes in blood vessels. Elevated blood pressure can strain the heart, leading to serious health complications if left uncontrolled.

Preventive Measures

- **Healthy Diet:** Seniors should adopt a heart-healthy diet rich in fruits, vegetables, whole grains, lean proteins, and low-fat dairy. Reducing sodium intake is crucial to managing blood pressure.
- **Regular Exercise:** The physical activity is a cornerstone of heart health. Seniors should engage in regular, age-appropriate exercise, such as walking, swimming, or yoga, to maintain cardiovascular fitness.
- **Weight Management:** Maintaining a healthy weight is essential. Weight loss, if necessary, can significantly improve heart health and reduce the risk of hypertension.
- **Stress Reduction:** Chronic stress can elevate blood pressure. Seniors should explore relaxation techniques like

meditation, deep breathing exercises, or hobbies to reduce stress levels.
- Limit Alcohol and Tobacco: Excessive alcohol consumption and smoking are detrimental to heart health. Seniors should consider quitting smoking and moderating alcohol intake.
- Regular Check-ups: Routine medical check-ups are vital for monitoring blood pressure, cholesterol levels, and overall heart health. Seniors should always follow their healthcare provider's recommendations.

Medication Management

In some cases, medication may be really necessary to control hypertension. Seniors should strictly adhere to their prescribed medication regimen and communicate any concerns or side effects to their healthcare provider.

Social Connections

Maintaining strong social connections is not only emotionally fulfilling but can also benefit heart health. Engaging in social activities and having a supportive network can reduce stress and promote overall well-being.

Heart health is paramount for seniors, and hypertension is a significant concern that must be addressed. By adopting a heart-healthy lifestyle, managing risk factors, and seeking regular medical care, seniors can protect their cardiovascular health and enjoy a fulfilling and active life in their golden years. It's never too late to prioritize your heart health and make positive changes for a longer, healthier life.

Weight Management for Seniors

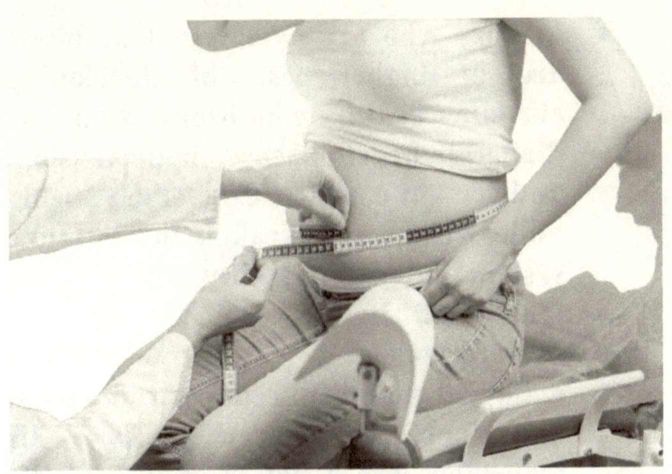

As individuals age, maintaining a very healthy weight becomes increasingly important for overall well-being. Weight management for seniors is not just about aesthetics; it plays a pivotal role in preventing and managing a range of health issues. In this comprehensive guide, we delve into the intricacies of weight management for seniors, offering insights, tips, and strategies for a healthier, happier life.

Understanding the Importance of Weight Management

- **Health Implications:**

- Seniors who are overweight or obese are at higher risk of developing chronic health conditions such as diabetes, heart disease, hypertension, and certain cancers. Conversely, being underweight can weaken the immune system and lead to frailty.
- Quality of Life:
- Maintaining a healthy weight enhances mobility, reduces joint pain, and increases energy levels. This translates into a better quality of life for seniors, enabling them to remain independent and engaged in activities they enjoy.

Factors Affecting Weight in Seniors

- Metabolism:
- Metabolism naturally slows with age, which means fewer calories are required. Seniors should adjust their calorie intake accordingly to avoid excess weight gain.
- Muscle Mass:

- Aging often leads to a decrease in muscle mass, which can lower the metabolic rate. Engaging in resistance training exercises can help counteract this loss.
- Hormonal Changes:
- Hormonal shifts, such as reduced growth hormone production, can contribute to fat accumulation. Consulting with a healthcare provider to address these changes is advisable.
- Medications:
- Certain medications can cause weight gain or loss. Seniors should communicate openly with their healthcare professionals about any concerns regarding medication side effects.

Tips for Effective Weight Management

- Balanced Diet:
- Emphasize on a diet rich in fruits, vegetables, lean proteins, whole grains, and healthy fats. Limit processed

foods such as, sugary snacks, and excessive salt intake.

- **Portion Control:**
- Seniors should be very mindful of portion sizes to prevent overeating. Smaller, frequent meals can help maintain energy levels and control hunger.
- **Hydration:**
- Staying well-hydrated is very crucial for overall health and can help control appetite. Seniors should aim to drink adequate water throughout the day.
- **Regular Exercise:**
- Engaging in a regular physical activity is essential for weight management. Activities like walking, swimming, yoga, and strength training can be tailored to suit individual capabilities.
- **Consult a Dietitian:**
- A registered dietitian can create personalized meal plans and offer dietary guidance tailored to a senior's specific needs and health conditions.
- **Supportive Community:**

- Joining support groups or participating in community fitness programs can provide motivation, social interaction, and encouragement on the weight management journey.
- Monitor Progress:
- Seniors should keep track of their weight, dietary habits, and physical activity. This self-awareness can help identify trends and make necessary adjustments.

Weight management for seniors is a multifaceted endeavor that encompasses physical, mental, and emotional well-being. By understanding the significance of maintaining a healthy weight, recognizing the factors that influence weight in later life, and adopting practical strategies, seniors can enjoy a fulfilling and active lifestyle. Remember, it's never too late to prioritize your health and make positive changes for a better tomorrow.

Joint and Bone Health

As we gracefully age, one of the paramount concerns that often takes center stage is the health of our joints and bones. These integral components of our musculoskeletal system serve as the scaffolding of our bodies, supporting our mobility, strength, and overall well-being. For seniors, preserving joint and bone health is not just about enhancing the quality of life, but also ensuring independence and longevity. In this comprehensive exploration, we delve into the essential aspects of joint and bone health for seniors.

Understanding the Aging Process

Before we embark on the journey of preserving joint and bone health, it is vital to grasp the changes that naturally occur as we age. As we grow older, our bones tend to lose density and become more brittle, making them susceptible to fractures. Simultaneously, the cartilage that cushions our joints begins to wear down, leading to stiffness and discomfort. These age-related changes can pave the way for conditions like osteoporosis and osteoarthritis, which can significantly affect an individual's quality of life.

The Role of Nutrition

Nutrition plays an instrumental role in maintaining joint and bone health. Seniors should focus on a diet rich in calcium and vitamin D, as these nutrients are pivotal for bone strength. Dairy products, leafy greens, and fortified foods are excellent sources of calcium, while exposure to sunlight helps the body synthesize vitamin D naturally.

Additionally, omega-3 fatty acids found in fish like salmon and walnuts possess anti-inflammatory properties, which can alleviate joint pain. Maintaining a balanced diet with an emphasis on whole grains, lean proteins, and fruits and vegetables provides the necessary nutrients for overall health.

Exercise for Stronger Joints and Bones

Regular physical activity is a cornerstone of joint and bone health for seniors. Weight-bearing exercises, such as walking, dancing, or even gardening, can help stimulate bone growth and maintain density. Strength training exercises, using resistance bands or light weights, enhance muscle strength, which, in turn, supports and protects the joints.

Flexibility and range-of-motion exercises, like yoga or tai chi, can alleviate stiffness and improve joint mobility. It's crucial to consult with a healthcare professional or a fitness expert to tailor an exercise regimen to individual needs and limitations.

Maintaining a Healthy Body Weight

Managing body weight is another crucial factor in safeguarding joint and bone health. Excess weight can exert additional pressure on the joints, particularly those in the knees and hips, increasing the risk of osteoarthritis. By maintaining a healthy weight through a balanced diet and regular exercise, seniors can reduce the strain on their joints and decrease the likelihood of developing joint-related problems.

Posture and Ergonomics

Proper posture and ergonomics play a subtle yet vital role in joint and bone health. Seniors should be mindful of their posture, especially when sitting for extended periods. Using ergonomic chairs and cushions can provide support to the spine and reduce the risk of back pain.

Regular Check-Ups and Medication

Regular medical check-ups are essential for monitoring joint and bone health. Seniors should discuss any joint pain, stiffness, or discomfort with their healthcare provider promptly. Early intervention can also help prevent the progression of conditions like osteoarthritis.

In some cases, medication or supplements may be prescribed to manage joint and bone health. It's crucial to follow medical advice diligently and report any side effects or concerns.

Joint and bone health is of paramount importance for seniors. Through a combination of proper nutrition, regular exercise, weight management, and attentive medical care, seniors can take proactive steps to preserve their joint and bone health. By embracing a holistic approach to aging gracefully, seniors can enjoy an active and fulfilling lifestyle, free from the limitations that joint and bone issues can impose. Remember, it's never too late to invest in your well-being and the longevity of your joints and bones.

Promoting Mental Well-Being for Seniors

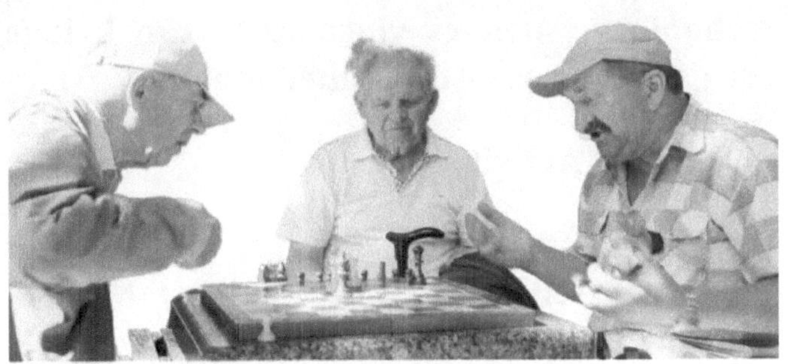

In the twilight years of life, mental well-being becomes an invaluable asset, often overshadowed by physical health concerns. As our loved ones and community members age, it is imperative to prioritize their emotional and psychological health. Here, we delve into the multifaceted approach to promoting mental well-being for seniors, recognizing the importance of this often overlooked aspect of their overall health.

1. Social Connection:

Loneliness and isolation can take a toll on a senior's mental health. Encouraging seniors to stay socially engaged is paramount. Regular family visits, community events, and senior centers can provide opportunities for meaningful interactions. Embracing technology, such as video calls, can bridge the gap for those with limited mobility.

2. Physical Activity:

The link between a physical activity and mental well-being is well-established. Encouraging seniors to stay active not only benefits their physical health but also releases endorphins, improving mood. Activities like gentle yoga, walking, or swimming can be tailored to individual capabilities.

3. Cognitive Stimulation:

Engaging the mind is crucial for seniors. Activities such as puzzles, reading, or learning a new skill can keep their cognitive faculties sharp and stave off cognitive decline. It's never too late to acquire new knowledge or explore a hobby.

4. Healthy Diet:

A balanced diet rich in nutrients can have a profound impact on mental well-being. Nutrient-dense foods, like fruits, vegetables, and whole grains, provide essential vitamins and minerals that support brain health. Adequate hydration is equally important.

5. Emotional Support:

Seniors may face various emotional challenges, including grief, loss of independence, or health issues. Providing a safe space for them to express their feelings and offering emotional support is vital. Professional counseling or therapy can be beneficial when needed.

6. Meaningful Activities:

Encourage seniors to pursue activities that bring them joy and a sense of purpose. This might include volunteering, participating in religious or spiritual practices, or engaging in creative endeavors like painting or writing.

7. Routine Healthcare:

Regular check-ups with healthcare professionals can detect and address any underlying physical or mental health issues promptly. Medication management is crucial for those with chronic conditions.

8. Mindfulness and Relaxation Techniques:

Teaching seniors mindfulness and relaxation techniques can help reduce stress and anxiety. Breathing exercises, meditation, or gentle stretching can promote a sense of calm and well-being.

9. Safety and Security:

Feeling safe in their environment is essential for seniors' mental well-being. Ensuring their home is hazard-free and implementing security measures can alleviate unnecessary worry.

10. Family and Community Involvement:

Families and communities play a pivotal role in seniors' mental well-being. Regular contact, listening, and involving them in family and community events can provide a strong sense of belonging and purpose.

Promoting mental well-being for seniors is a holistic endeavor that encompasses physical, emotional, social, and cognitive aspects of their lives. By recognizing the importance of mental health in aging individuals and implementing these strategies, we can enhance the quality of life for our seniors, allowing them to age gracefully and with the happiness and fulfillment they deserve.

Chapter 6: Staying Active and Fit

The Importance of Senior Fitness

Low-Impact Exercises for Seniors

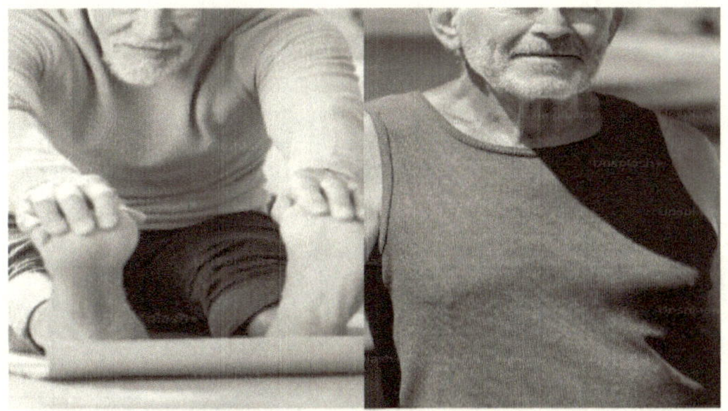

Aging gracefully is a goal that many seniors aspire to achieve, and maintaining an active lifestyle is a crucial component of that journey.

While high-intensity workouts may have their place in fitness, low-impact exercises emerge as the unsung heroes for seniors, offering a plethora of benefits without putting undue stress on aging joints and muscles. In this comprehensive guide, we delve into the world of low-impact exercises for seniors, exploring the profound impact they can have on physical and mental well-being.

The Importance of Low-Impact Exercises

As the years advance, the body undergoes inevitable changes, including reduced bone density, muscle mass, and joint flexibility. The fear of injury or discomfort can often discourage seniors from engaging in physical activity. This is where low-impact exercises shine, as they provide a gentle, yet effective, way to combat these age-related challenges.

Gentle Aerobics: Walking and Swimming

Walking, the simplest form of exercise, is a powerhouse for seniors. It improves cardiovascular health, enhances bone density, and can be tailored to individual fitness levels. Regular strolls in the park or around the neighborhood not only keep the heart pumping but also offer an opportunity to enjoy the outdoors and socialize.

For those who seek a full-body workout with minimal joint strain, swimming is a fantastic choice. The buoyancy of water reduces the impact on joints while engaging all major muscle groups. Whether it's a leisurely swim or water aerobics, seniors can build strength, flexibility, and endurance in a soothing aquatic environment.

Flexibility and Balance: Yoga and Tai Chi

Flexibility and balance are crucial aspects of senior fitness. Yoga and Tai Chi are low-impact exercises that excel in these domains. Yoga's gentle stretching and breathing techniques promote flexibility, muscle tone, and relaxation. Tai Chi, often described as "meditation in motion," enhances balance and coordination, reducing the risk of falls.

Strength Training: Resistance Bands and Bodyweight Exercises

Preserving muscle mass is essential as we age, and strength training plays a pivotal role. Seniors can opt for resistance band exercises, which provide gradual resistance without the need for heavy weights. Bodyweight exercises such as squats, leg raises, and push-ups can also be modified to suit individual abilities, strengthening muscles and bones over time.

Mind-Body Connection: Pilates and Mindfulness

Low-impact exercises aren't just about physical health; they also nurture the mind-body connection. Pilates, with its focus on core strength, flexibility, and controlled movements, improves posture and reduces the risk of back pain. Additionally, practicing mindfulness through meditation or deep breathing exercises can alleviate stress and enhance mental well-being.

Tailoring the Routine

One of the strengths of low-impact exercises is their adaptability. Seniors can customize their routines to match their fitness levels, preferences, and any existing health conditions. Consulting with a healthcare professional or a certified fitness trainer is advised to ensure a safe and effective exercise program.

The Journey Towards Wellness

Low-impact exercises for seniors open a gateway to a healthier, more vibrant life in the golden years. They are not merely physical activities but holistic practices that nurture the body and mind. By incorporating these exercises into their daily routines, seniors can savor the joys of staying active, enjoying improved mobility, and sowing the seeds of longevity. Remember, age is but a number, and with the right approach to fitness, it can be accompanied by a rich tapestry of health and vitality.

Yoga and Stretching for Flexibility

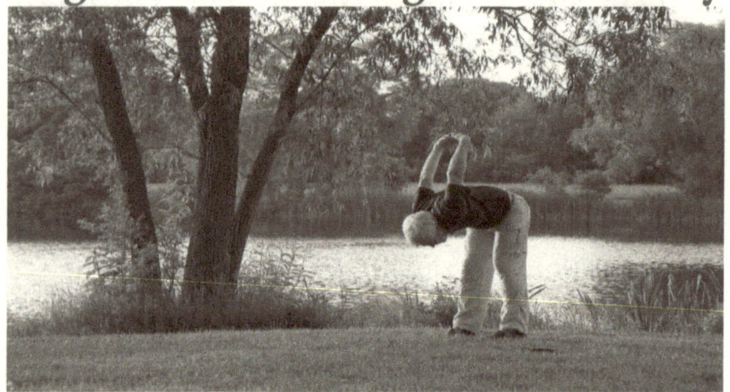

As we journey through the tapestry of life, the golden years often beckon with the promise of relaxation and reflection. However, for many seniors, this phase can be marred by the discomfort of stiff joints and diminished flexibility. Thankfully, the ancient practice of yoga, coupled with targeted stretching exercises, offers a pathway towards reclaiming and maintaining flexibility, vitality, and overall well-being in the twilight years.

Yoga, with its roots stretching back thousands of years in India, is a holistic discipline that blends physical postures, controlled breathing, and meditation. For seniors, it's a gentle yet profoundly effective way to enhance flexibility, strength, and balance. The beauty of yoga lies in its adaptability; poses can be modified to suit individual needs and abilities, making it an inclusive practice for all ages.

One of the primary benefits of yoga is its impact on flexibility. Seniors often face challenges with joint stiffness and reduced range of motion due to natural aging processes. Yoga asanas (postures) gently coax the body into various positions, targeting muscle groups and joints that may have become dormant over time. Regular practice helps to lengthen and strengthen muscles, thereby improving flexibility.

Gentle stretches and yoga poses like the Cat-Cow, Downward Dog, and Child's Pose are particularly beneficial for seniors. These poses elongate the spine, increase blood flow to the muscles, and promote a sense of relaxation and ease. Moreover, yoga encourages a mindful connection between the body and the breath, fostering greater awareness of physical sensations and helping seniors avoid pushing themselves too hard, which could lead to injury.

In addition to yoga, targeted stretching exercises are essential in promoting flexibility for seniors. These stretches can target specific muscle groups, addressing common issues like tight hamstrings, stiff shoulders, and inflexible hips. A consistent stretching routine can alleviate discomfort and improve daily activities such as bending down to tie shoelaces or reaching for items on high shelves.

When embarking on a journey to enhance flexibility through yoga and stretching, seniors should consider a few key principles:

- Consistency: Regular practice is key to reaping the benefits of yoga and stretching.Get started slowly and gradually build up your practice over time.
- Safety: Listen to your body and practice within your comfort zone.

Avoid overstretching or pushing yourself too hard to prevent injury.

- Variety: Incorporate a variety of poses and stretches to target different muscle groups and maintain a well-rounded flexibility routine.
- Breath Awareness: Pay attention to your breath while practicing yoga and stretching. Deep, controlled breaths can help relax muscles and deepen stretches.
- Seek Guidance: If you're new to yoga or have specific health concerns, consider working with a certified yoga instructor or physical therapist who can tailor a practice to your needs.

Yoga and stretching offer a powerful antidote to the challenges of aging. They provide seniors with a means to regain and maintain flexibility, fostering not only physical well-being but also mental and emotional balance. Through consistent practice, individuals can gracefully navigate the journey of aging, embracing each day with vitality, flexibility, and a sense of inner peace.

Incorporating Physical Activity into Daily Life.

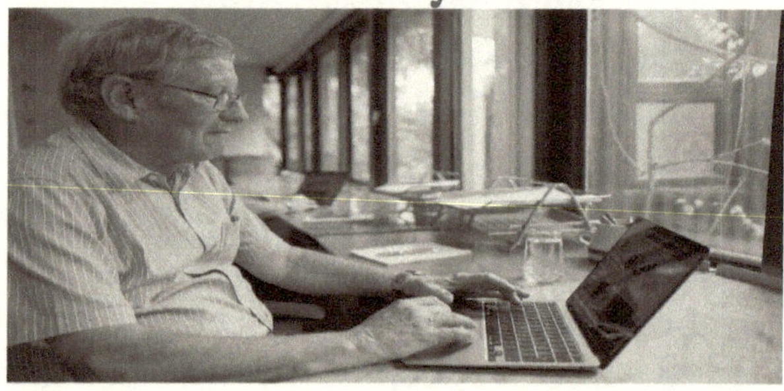

As we gracefully age, it becomes increasingly important to prioritize our physical well-being. One of the key pillars of a healthy lifestyle for seniors is regular physical activity. Contrary to the misconception that age hinders physical engagement, incorporating exercise into daily life can be both enjoyable and immensely beneficial for seniors. In this comprehensive guide, we explore the numerous ways in which seniors can embrace physical activity as an integral part of their daily routines.

Understanding the Importance of Physical Activity for Seniors

Before delving into specific activities, it's crucial to grasp the significance of physical activity for seniors. Engaging in regular exercise offers a plethora of advantages, ranging from improved mobility and balance to enhanced mental well-being. It also helps reduce the risk of chronic illnesses such as heart disease, diabetes, and osteoporosis. By staying active, seniors can maintain their independence and overall quality of life.

Tailoring Activities to Individual Needs and Abilities

The first step in incorporating physical activities into daily life for seniors is recognizing that one size does not fit all. Every individual is unique, and physical activities should be tailored to one's specific needs and abilities. It's essential to consult with a healthcare provider or a fitness professional to determine the most suitable exercises and intensity levels based on individual health conditions and limitations.

Exploring Low-Impact Exercises

Low-impact exercises are gentle on the joints and are excellent choices for seniors. Walking, swimming, and cycling are low-impact activities that provide cardiovascular benefits without subjecting the body to excessive stress. Water aerobics, in particular, is an enjoyable way to improve strength and flexibility while being easy on the joints.

Strength Training for Healthy Aging

Maintaining muscle mass is essential for seniors as it helps prevent falls and supports overall mobility. Incorporating strength training exercises, such as resistance band exercises, bodyweight squats, and light weightlifting, can enhance muscle tone and bone density. These activities can be performed at home or in a supervised gym setting.

Flexibility and Balance Exercises

Seniors can greatly benefit from exercises that improve flexibility and balance. Yoga and tai chi are excellent options that promote relaxation, enhance balance, and increase joint mobility. These mind-body practices also help reduce stress and contribute to better mental health.

Staying Social and Active

Physical activity need not be a solitary pursuit. Seniors can engage in group activities like dance classes, group walks, or even joining a local sports club. These social interactions not only promote physical health but also provide a sense of community and emotional well-being.

Incorporating Activity into Daily Routine

Making physical activity a part of daily life requires a proactive approach. Seniors can start by setting achievable goals and gradually increasing their activity levels. Activities like gardening, taking the stairs instead of the elevator, or doing household chores can all contribute to daily exercise.

Safety First

Safety should always be a top priority. Seniors should wear appropriate footwear, stay hydrated, and pay attention to their bodies. If any exercise causes pain or discomfort, it's important to stop immediately and consult with a healthcare professional.

Incorporating physical activities into daily life for seniors is a holistic approach to healthy aging. By customizing activities to individual needs, embracing low-impact exercises, and fostering social connections, seniors can enjoy the numerous benefits of staying active. It's never too late to embark on a journey toward better health and well-being, and with the right guidance and determination, seniors can lead fulfilling lives filled with vitality and vigor. Remember, the key is to start small, stay consistent, and savor the journey towards a healthier, happier, and more active senior life.

Chapter 7: Lifestyle and Longevity

Stress Reduction and Relaxation Techniques

Sleep and Senior Health

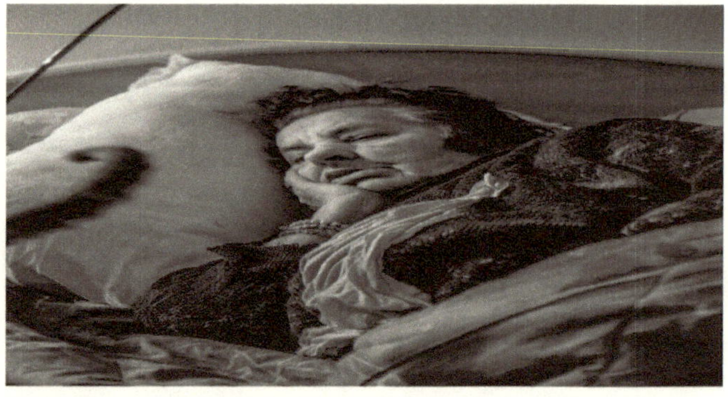

Sleep is a fundamental aspect of human life, one that becomes increasingly critical as we age. In the context of senior health, it's not merely a luxury; it's a lifeline to overall well-being and vitality. This powerful connection between sleep and senior health is often underestimated, but its impact is profound,

influencing both physical and mental aspects of aging.

The Importance of Sleep

Sleep can be described as the body's natural healer, and for good reason. It is during sleep that our bodies engage in repair and restoration processes that are crucial for maintaining health. From a physiological standpoint, sleep plays a pivotal role in regulating various bodily functions, including metabolism, immune system function, and hormonal balance.

For seniors, who may already be dealing with age-related health issues, the quality and quantity of sleep become even more crucial. Unfortunately, many seniors experience sleep disturbances, which can lead to a vicious cycle of health decline. It's imperative to understand the implications of poor sleep on senior health to appreciate the urgency of addressing this issue.

The Impact on Physical Health

- **Cardiovascular Health:** Sleep disturbances are associated with an increased risk of cardiovascular diseases, such as hypertension, stroke, and heart disease. Seniors who consistently experience poor sleep are more vulnerable to these life-threatening conditions.
- **Immune Function:** A robust immune system is essential for seniors, especially in the face of infections and diseases. Inadequate sleep weakens immune function, making seniors more susceptible to illnesses.
- **Metabolic Health:** Sleep is intricately linked to metabolic health. Sleep deprivation can lead to weight gain and insulin resistance, increasing the risk of diabetes and obesity, both of which are significant concerns for seniors.
- **Pain Management:** Seniors often grapple with chronic pain conditions. Sleep disturbances can exacerbate pain perception, making it more challenging to manage discomfort.

The Impact on Mental Health

- **Cognitive Decline: Adequate sleep is vital for cognitive function. Seniors who don't get enough sleep are at a higher risk of cognitive decline, including memory problems and an increased likelihood of developing conditions like Alzheimer's disease.**
- **Mood Disorders: Sleep and mental health are deeply interconnected. Poor sleep can lead to depression and anxiety, which are prevalent among seniors. Conversely, these conditions can also disrupt sleep patterns.**
- **Quality of Life: A lack of sleep can significantly reduce one's overall quality of life. Seniors who consistently struggle with sleep may experience reduced motivation, social withdrawal, and a diminished sense of well-being.**

Strategies for Improving Sleep in Seniors

- **Establish a Routine: Consistency is key. Encourage seniors to go to bed**

and wake up at the same time every day, even on weekends.
- **Create a Comfortable Sleep Environment: Ensure the bedroom is very conducive to sleep by keeping it in a dark, quiet, and at a comfortable temperature.**
- **Limit Screen Time: Reduce exposure to screens (phones, TVs, computers) before bedtime, as the blue light emitted can interfere with the body's natural sleep-wake cycle.**
- **Promote Relaxation: Encourage relaxation techniques such as meditation, deep breathing, or gentle stretching exercises to help seniors wind down before bedtime.**
- **Diet and Exercise: A balanced diet and regular physical activity can promote better sleep. However, avoid heavy meals and strenuous exercise close to bedtime.**

Sleep is an indispensable pillar of senior health. Recognizing the intricate connection between sleep and overall well-being is the

first step toward improving the health and quality of life for seniors. By implementing strategies to enhance sleep quality, we can empower our aging population to age gracefully, maintaining both their physical and mental vitality.

Social Engagement and Mental Stimulation

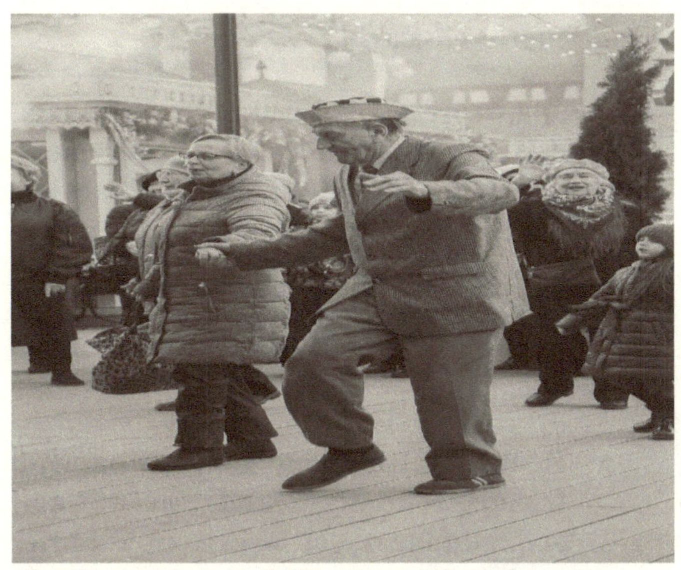

In the tapestry of life, the senior years are a unique and precious thread. As individuals transition into this phase, the importance of social engagement and mental stimulation takes center stage. This period offers an opportunity not only for relaxation but also for continued growth, learning, and emotional well-being. In this exploration, we delve into the profound impact of social interaction and cognitive engagement on the lives of seniors.

Social Engagement: The Lifeline of Emotional Well-Being

The aging process often comes hand in hand with certain life changes – retirement, children leaving the nest, and sometimes the loss of loved ones. These transitions can lead to feelings of isolation and loneliness, which can have detrimental effects on one's mental and physical health. This is where social engagement emerges as a lifeline.

- **Reducing Isolation:** Connecting with friends, family, and even new acquaintances can serve as a buffer against isolation. Regular interactions can provide a sense of belonging and

purpose that is essential for emotional well-being.

- **Enhancing Emotional Resilience: Sharing stories, experiences, and laughter with others can help seniors cope with life's challenges. It provides an outlet for emotions and fosters emotional resilience.**
- **Stimulating Cognitive Functions: Engaging in conversations, debates, or even playing board games can stimulate cognitive functions, keeping the mind agile and alert. These interactions are like a workout for the brain, preventing cognitive decline.**
- **Boosting Self-Esteem: Social engagement provides opportunities to share wisdom and knowledge gained over a lifetime. Seniors' contributions to conversations and activities can boost their self-esteem and sense of accomplishment.**

Mental Stimulation: The Fountain of Youth for the Mind

As the body ages, so does the brain. Mental stimulation is the key to keeping this vital organ sharp and active. It involves activities that challenge cognitive abilities, keeping the brain engaged and resilient.

- **Learning New Skills:** It's never too late to acquire new skills. Whether it's picking up a musical instrument, learning a new language, or taking up painting, these endeavors not only stimulate the mind but also instill a sense of achievement.
- **Reading and Problem Solving:** Reading regularly and engaging in puzzles, crosswords, or Sudoku puzzles can maintain and even enhance cognitive abilities. These activities require focus, memory, and problem-solving skills.
- **Technology and Digital Literacy:** Embracing technology can open up new avenues for mental stimulation. Seniors can explore the world of smartphones, tablets, and computers

to stay connected and access a wealth of information.

- **Physical Exercise:** It's worth mentioning that physical exercise isn't just beneficial for the body; it also enhances mental health. Regular physical activity can improve mood, reduce stress, and boost cognitive functions.

The senior years are a chapter of life filled with potential and opportunity. Social engagement and mental stimulation are not just luxuries but necessities for seniors to thrive emotionally and cognitively. These activities not only enrich their lives but also contribute to a vibrant, resilient, and fulfilling later life. As we honor and cherish our seniors, let us also empower them to continue growing, learning, and connecting, for they are the keepers of wisdom and the treasures of our society.

Aging Gracefully with the Weight Loss Diet

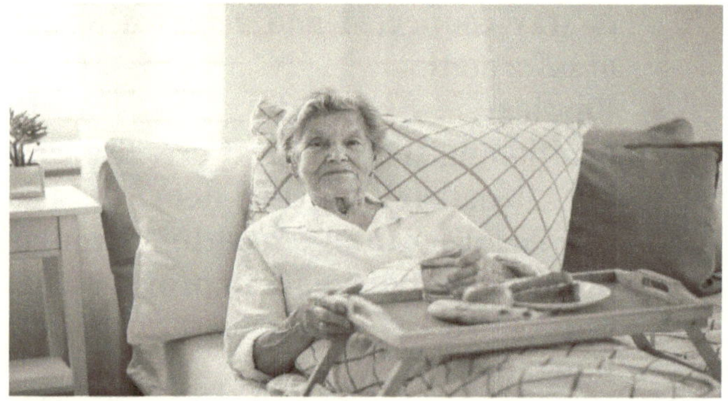

Aging is an inevitable part of life, but how we age can be greatly influenced by our lifestyle choices, particularly when it comes to nutrition. For seniors seeking to embrace their golden years with vigor and vitality, the Weight Loss Diet offers a compelling approach to aging gracefully. This dietary plan, rooted in balanced nutrition and mindful eating, not only supports weight management but also promotes overall health and well-being.

The Essence of Aging Gracefully

Aging gracefully is about more than just looking good on the surface; it's about feeling your best from the inside out. The Weight

Loss Diet recognizes this fundamental truth and aims to empower seniors to live their fullest lives as they age. It places emphasis on long-term health rather than quick fixes, fostering a sustainable and holistic approach to well-being.

Balanced Nutrition as the Foundation

At the core of the Weight Loss Diet is a commitment to balanced nutrition. Seniors are encouraged to consume a variety of whole foods, including lean proteins, whole grains, fresh fruits, and vegetables. These nutrient-dense choices provide essential vitamins and minerals, supporting optimal bodily functions and helping to combat age-related health concerns.

The Weight Loss Diet's Emphasis on Blood Sugar Management

One of the standout features of the Weight Loss Diet is its emphasis on blood sugar management. This is particularly significant for seniors, as fluctuating blood sugar levels can lead to various health issues, including diabetes and heart disease. The diet's focus on low-glycemic foods helps stabilize blood sugar levels, reducing the risk of these conditions and promoting the overall health.

Healthy Fats and Aging Brain

Aging often brings concerns about cognitive decline, but the Weight Loss Diet has an answer to that as well. By incorporating healthy fats like avocados, nuts, and olive oil, seniors can nourish their brains with essential nutrients that support memory and cognitive function. This is a powerful way to age gracefully by preserving mental clarity and sharpness.

Portion Control and Mindful Eating

Portion control is to be a cornerstone of the Weight Loss Diet. Seniors are encouraged to listen to their bodies and eat mindfully, savoring each bite. This practice not only helps with weight management but also fosters a deeper connection with food, promoting better digestion and satisfaction.

Exercise and Mobility

Aging gracefully isn't just about diet; it's also about maintaining physical vitality. The Weight Loss Diet recognizes this and encourages seniors to incorporate regular exercise into their routine. This can be tailored to individual fitness levels and needs, ensuring that seniors stay active and mobile as they age.

Embracing Positive Lifestyle Changes

Aging gracefully with the weight Loss Diet is not just about what you eat; it's a holistic lifestyle approach. It's about prioritizing self-care, getting enough rest, managing stress, and nurturing social connections. These elements are essential for emotional and mental well-being, which are equally important in the journey of graceful aging.

This is a journey that extends beyond physical appearance. It's about cultivating a rich and fulfilling life as you age, one where health, vitality, and happiness take center stage. By prioritizing balanced nutrition, blood sugar management, mindful eating, and overall well-being, seniors can embark on this journey with confidence, knowing that they have the tools to make the most of their golden years. It's a testament to the power of lifestyle choices in shaping our destinies, proving that age is just a number when you nourish your body and soul with care and intention.

Chapter 8: Conclusion

Your Path to Prolonged Healthy Living.

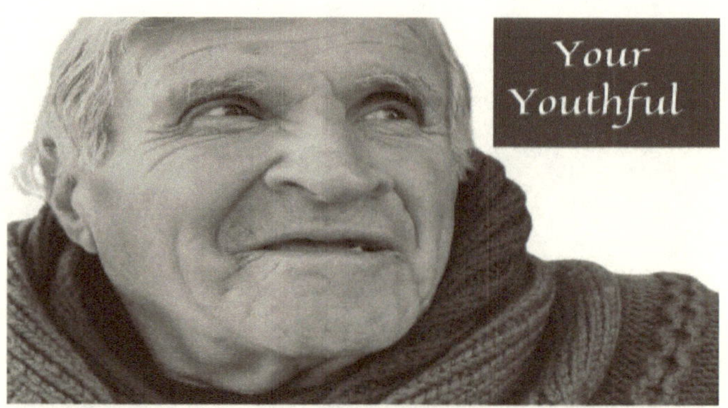

comprehensive guide on how you can embark on your own path to a long and healthy life.

1. Mindful Nutrition: The foundation of a healthy life begins with what we put into our bodies. A balanced and nutritious diet is key.

Focus on a whole, unprocessed foods like fruits, vegetables, lean proteins, whole grains, and healthy fats. Limit sugar and processed foods, and practice portion control.

2. Hydration: Water is the elixir of life. Making sure to stay adequately hydrated is crucial for various bodily functions. Aim to drink plenty of water throughout the day, and consider herbal teas or infused water for added flavor and benefits.

3. Regular Exercise: Inlcude physical activity into your daily routine. Whether it's a brisk walk, yoga, weight training, or any other form of exercise you enjoy, consistency is key. Aim for at least 150 minutes of moderate-intensity exercise per week.

4. Quality Sleep: Prioritize sleep as a cornerstone of good health. Be aiming for 7-9 hours of restful sleep each night. Create a calming bedtime routine, avoid screens before sleep, and maintain a consistent sleep schedule.

5. Stress Management: Chronic stress can have detrimental effects on your health. Practice stress-reduction techniques such as meditation, deep breathing exercises, mindfulness, or hobbies that bring you joy.

6. Regular Check-ups: Don't neglect regular health check-ups and screenings. Early detection of health issues can be a lifesaver. Be proactive in managing your health by scheduling routine appointments with your healthcare provider.

7. Social Connections: Nurturing meaningful relationships and a strong social support network can positively impact mental and emotional well-being. Engage in social activities, connect with loved ones, and seek support when needed.

8. Mental Well-being: Prioritize mental health just as you would physical health. Seek professional help if you're facing challenges like anxiety, depression, or other mental health issues. Practice self-compassion and self-care.

9. **Avoid Harmful Habits:** Steer clear of smoking, excessive alcohol consumption, and recreational drug use. These habits can significantly shorten your lifespan and diminish your quality of life.

10. **Lifelong Learning:** Keep your mind engaged and active. Be in continuous search of opportunities for learning and personal growth. This can include reading, taking courses, pursuing hobbies, or acquiring new skills.

11. **Environmental Awareness:** Be mindful of the environment you live in. Reduce exposure to pollutants, toxins, and harmful chemicals. Opt for sustainable practices that not only benefit your health but also the planet.

12. **Purpose and Passion:** Find meaning and purpose in your life. Pursue activities and passions that ignite your soul and give you a reason to wake up each day with enthusiasm.

13. **Adaptability:** Life is unpredictable. Cultivate resilience and adaptability.

Embrace change and navigate challenges with a positive mindset.

14. Balanced Work-Life: Achieving a work-life balance is essential for overall well-being. Avoid overworking and prioritize leisure time, family, and personal pursuits.

15. Gratitude: Practice gratitude daily. Recognize and appreciate the blessings in your life, as this fosters a positive outlook and enhances mental and emotional health.

Remember, the path to prolonged healthy living is not a destination but a lifelong journey. Small, consistent choices made every day can accumulate into a life filled with vitality, happiness, and longevity. It's never too late to start, so take that first step today on your journey to a healthier, happier you.